Food Makes Me Happy

(and that's my problem!)

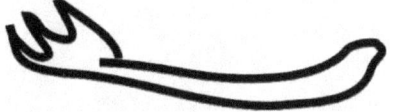

Food Makes Me Happy

(and that's my problem!)

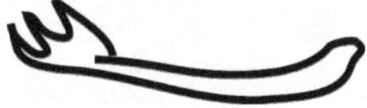

By Michael Sortino

ISBN 1440476349 (trade pbk.)

To my wonderful wife and children, who make me want to be around a whole heck of a lot longer.

Acknowledgements

In addition to my precious wife and kids, I'd like to thank my parents, brother, sisters, in-laws, and friends (thanks Frank for the amazing artwork!) for all your encouragement, example and support through the years.

I'd especially like to thank my Maker for making me, for making food, and for actually making a pretty darn good way for the two of us to get along!

Table of Contents

"Thou shouldst eat to live; not live to eat."
- Socrates

"Part of the secret of success in life is to eat what you like and let the food fight it out inside."
- Mark Twain

Disclaimer

Anyone reading this book expecting to learn how to lose thirty to forty pounds in two weeks or less, has come to the wrong place. I don't have any miracle cure, nor am I attempting to persuade anyone which diet out there is the best or the worst.

I don't have a PhD. I'm not a body-builder or a magazine model. I'm just an average, American man who's noticed something about this whole weight-watching phenomenon that no one seems to want to talk about. Maybe it's because the advice I have to give, you can't package and sell in a bottle—that's not to say you won't see me on an infomercial three months after reading this, trying to do just that. Hey, I'm trying to support a family of six, here. I'm not above anything.

This brings up another <u>important note</u>: I tend to joke around quite a bit, so be careful you don't take all that you read here at face value. I figure, if you can't laugh at your life, you're not really living it.

So, what follows is, hopefully, a refreshing and insightful look at why we tend to gain weight when we want to lose it, and how we can put our lives on a healthy track that will inevitably lead to looking and feeling the way we were meant to look and feel.

Enjoy! And, by the way, this book is completely edible, so, at bare minimum, if you get anything out of it, it'll be a nice, fiber-rich meal! See important note, above.

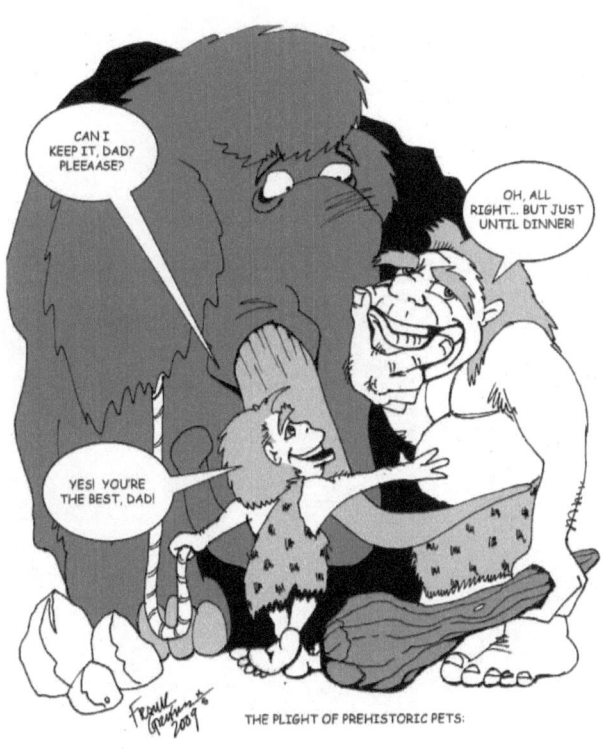

THE PLIGHT OF PREHISTORIC PETS:

In the Beginning . . . there was the Pizza Hoagie
(A brief treatment on the history of food)

From the moment man had his first craving for half-baked Mammoth leg, one of the most intimate, thought about, written about and universally participated in relationships began: that is, the human being and that oftentimes delectable, sometimes detestable and hopefully digestible thing we all like to call food.

Now, man basically hunted or grew his food in the beginning. There were no pesticides or preservatives to worry about, let alone things called trans fatty acids. Of course, there were no refrigerators either, or microwaves; and concerns about Sal manila would've, at the most, brought up a discussion of some distant relative in the Philippines.

Food was cherished, though, for two reasons: People understood early on that they needed it to live, and it was not something you could always depend on being around. What if the hunters had a bad week? What if there was a drought? Food had to last and it could not, under any circumstances, be wasted. In fact, every part of an animal killed in the hunt was used for something, and a lot of that was food.

Little Tondor, on his birthday, was probably thrilled to get a sloth bladder. He could have fun with it for the day but, by nightfall, I'm sure he had to fork that thing over for the family meal. He probably knew better than to complain or argue. It was simply understood. Food equaled survival.

It only follows that overeating was considered a crime. If someone, at the end of a meal said, "You know, that saber-tooth tripe was just so darn good, I think I'll have some more," they would have been clubbed, unanimously.

Moving a bit forward in time, you met the opposite extreme with the Romans. You've heard of the vomitoriums, I'm sure. These were handy little bowl-shaped repositories kept by the table during meal time for the elite, so that, if they ran out of space for the sixteenth entrée, they could simply make room for more.

Imagine being the poor slaves that had to be on V-duty? Can you just hear the discussion in the kitchen?

"I can't take this anymore. If I have to dump out another half-digested—I'm not going back in there."

"If you don't, Syrius, they'll throw you to the lions."

"We'll at least the lions know when to stop. I'd rather take my chances with them. I'm serious."

[6]

"I, uh, know. We met earlier, remember?"

I'm surprised someone hasn't tried to bring those lovely items back into the mainstream marketplace. They could come in different shapes and sizes and colors. There could be the stainless steel, company lunch room one, all the way up to the gold-trimmed fancy china piece that you brought out for special occasions.

Can't you see them fitting right in to most homes in well-off countries?

"Honey, Aunt Edna's done with her lamb chops. Can you pass her the vomitorium?"

"She's got her own strapped to the bottom of her chair, dear."

"No, no. She broke through that chair at lunch."

"Oh, that's right."

Thanksgiving would no longer be a day where the turkeys had the last laugh. "Yes, we're so thankful for all the food we have. Let's stuff ourselves until we nearly pop and wish we were never born." (For more on this, see Chapter 8—Holidays are Not Evil).

Okay, in all seriousness, most of us know that the Romans passed this practice all the way down to present day. Although, in most cultures, it is a covert action taken by those who have convinced themselves they will never be thin enough and that, whatever food goes into them in excess of their diseased perception of what is right, must come out. It is a growing epidemic among women and men alike, a disease that must be acknowledged and treated, and a tragedy that we'll get into more, later in the book.

Coming into the Renaissance, we find a stance on the human figure that is curious, if not downright preposterous to those today who buy into the current fashion mindset. In a nutshell, portly was "in."

Women were not considered attractive unless they had some meat on their bones, and a good deal of it. We see it portrayed in the art work. Why do you think the Mona Lisa's got that sly little smile on? She's thinking, "I can eat all I want and not have to worry about it. Ha. Ha. Pass the pudding."

> *Food for Thought:*
> *Do I pay too much attention to what the current trend or magazine people say about how I should look?*

Today's supermodels would have been super duds back then. If a man couldn't count on his woman to stop a runaway horse cart with her left thigh, she was not worth bothering with.

With the Industrial Revolution came one of the greatest food inventions the world has ever seen, the sandwich. Think about it. People had to man the machines, meet those shipping deadlines. There wasn't time to sit down with a knife and fork and slop up some Yorkshire minced meat pie.

The sandwich, which not coincidentally came from England, the same place the modern era emerged from, was invented so that the average worker could eat with one hand and still operate standard factory equipment with the other.

This was one of the reasons the Pilgrims took off for the Americas. See, these people were all about sit-down meals with your family, among other things, of course. When they landed on Plymouth Rock, they were hungry, as you know. Food had run out, people were getting scurvy and the like. Still, I bet if a convoy of Native Americans greeted them on the shoreline with an offering of turkey sandwiches, they would have flat out rejected them.

That's why, when Thanksgiving rolled around, they said, "*This* is how it's done. Let me tell you!" And, they spread the whole thing out with plates for every type of food. Little did they know that America would become the fast food capital of the world someday. Talk about historical irony. Go on, talk about it! Put the book down, now, and turn to the person next to you to discuss just how darn ironic that is, in a historical sense!

Sorry, I get a little passionate at times.

Now, it was tough going in the early days of the Colonies. Again, history repeats itself. Just like in any survival situation, food was cherished and not generally abused. One could easily see from the Boston Tea Party incident, where Americans raided a newly arrived shipment of tea from the Motherland and dumped it into Boston's harbor, just how hungry these people were.

"Great Scott! They've sent us tea! Tea, of all things!" you could hear one of the instigators saying. "That stuff is going overboard, I tell you! Over! Board!"

Now, if they had included a few crates of biscuits on that ship, we may have seen a different outcome. Not with the formation of the country, mind you. There was that whole taxation without representation thing, you know. But, basically that, too, boiled down to the fact that the colonists were tired of handing over their food money without having any say in their own destiny.

If Thomas Jefferson could've really written what was on most people's minds, the Declaration of Independence would've started out something more like this: We hold these truths to be self-evident, that all men are created equal. So, why should King Georgey Porgey over there be shoving his face at every meal when we can barely scrape together a corn chowder on a good Tuesday?"

Food for Thought: Just because we're free to eat an entire chocolate cake in one sitting, does it mean we should?

Our freedom was purchased with a heavy price tag (and is still maintained by one, I know, and truly appreciate) but I'm going to conclude this time travel chapter with a troubling, if not controversial question: Has it done us more harm than good? Just in the category of food, alone. Reflect on this: As the country grew in prosperity and power, so did the waistline of its average citizen. The easier it was to get food, the more, I believe, it became and has become taken for granted. I'm not saying bring back the good old days of the Empire, mind you. And, I'm all about freedom, for sure. It's just nothing we should take lightly, that's all.

And, that's all for now on that. I think it's good to look at where our relationship with food began and how it's progressed through the ages. I apologize that it was from an entirely Western point of view. This could not be helped for two reasons: One, it is my own personal vantage point and, two, it's where all of my hardcore research and rock-solid, fact-finding energy has been spent. Yes, you can chuckle at that.

Now, in the next chapter, I'm going to stray a little bit from historical fact to share about my own personal relationship with food.

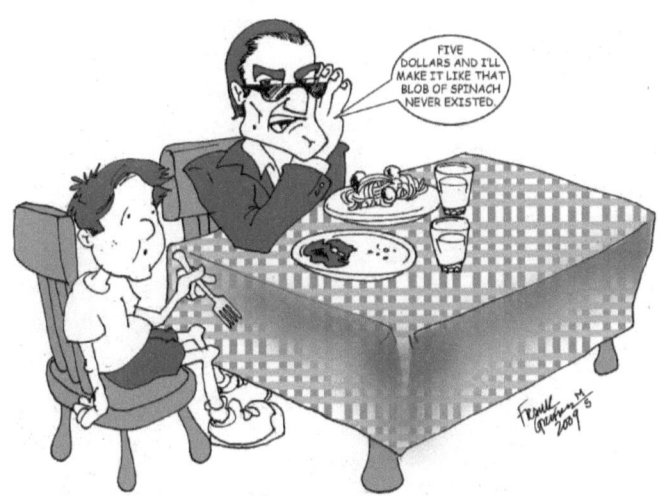

UNCLE GUIDO MAKES BOBBY AN OFFER HE CAN'T REFUSE...

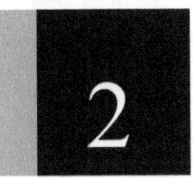

Food is Life
(Confessions of a once and future chubby Italian-American)

Having grown up in an Italian American family, I will say one thing: We put food in its rightful place . . . our mouths.

A lot of people think that, because Italians are always saying, "Mangia! Mangia! (Eat! Eat!)," they have an unhealthy perspective on food. Not so. Well, at least not entirely so. Italians are human just like everyone else, though some of my relatives may tell you there's a touch of superhuman in our heritage (a viewpoint which primarily comes from the fact that we are able to make our own pasta from scratch).

The memories I have of family life are garnished heavily with food: Raviolis, baked ziti, eggplant parmesan, meatballs, ricotta sandwiches. These are some of the favorites I can remember. And, of course, pasta. Pasta. Pasta. Pasta.

It's no small wonder that the proponents of the low-carb diet are not Italian. Pasta was a staple in our home. (Yes, I often used it to hold homework pages together.) As kids, we went from asking, "Ma, what are we having for dinner?" to "Ma, we're having pasta and *what* for dinner?"

Man, I loved pasta. I could eat it at every meal. In fact, I may start a line of breakfast cereals for Italian kids: Fruity Pastas! Or, Captain Pasta! Then, of course, you could have Honey Nut Pastios.

> **Food for Thought:**
> *How does it make me feel when I do something good for someone else?*

When we went to our grandmother's house, it didn't matter what time of day it was, she could have a steaming bowl of macaroni and red sauce poised under your nose in under two minutes flat. This, as she would readily admit, was one of her primary purposes in life. I could see, just like with my own mother, it gave her great satisfaction to see her family fed, and fed well.

A byproduct of this, however, was the guilt that came along with turning down a maternal family member who offered you food. You had this sinking gut feeling that such a denial was a direct insult to their very core, a cut-down that could very well crush them. So, when Aunt Frances offered you another cannoli, you tried hard to swallow the third one you were working on, and you said, "Yef, fank-oo."

You might ask, how long could this possibly go on? Usually until one of us passed out. And, forget about it, if we went to Italy! Sheez! It was an international incident if we left the table within an hour. We had to learn very quickly how to say, "I'm full," in Italian, and, "Seriously, I'm going to die if I eat another bite!" That was a handy phrase as well.

Awards were handed out for being good eaters. My brother, sisters and I were sources of pride to our parents, sure, on many other fine points, but right up there was eating. Obviously, it's so much more pleasant when a kid chews and swallows his food rather than throws it in your face in front of company, but this went farther than that. You could feel it deep within, the honor you brought the family by licking the plate clean.

And, yes, I may be exaggerating in retrospect, but all I'm saying is that I am the all-time greatest Ricotta and pasta-eating champion and, if any of my siblings think they can to take me on, I'm ready! Bring it on! Name the kitchen and sauce type, and I'm there!

The point I'm making is that, from early on, we were taught to believe that eating the food put in front of you was a very important thing to do. In some cases, it did come down to survival. Especially, with me and avocados. To this day, I can't stomach them. Well, actually, I could probably stomach them if I could just get them in there without having to go through the mouth part. I don't know what it is. Maybe it's because they're slimy, green, and taste like alien brains, but I had a great aversion to these confused, fruit/vegetable/all-around-disturbing items.

However, I knew that if I didn't finish them, I would be in big trouble. Basically, I was chained to the table until I either a) gulped them down after scalding my taste buds with boiling water and then chasing them down with any other liquid, b) lost a week's allowance pawning them off on another sibling, or c) finished them like a real man. Needless to say, option "c" rarely happened.

"It's good for you!" was the phrase I would get the most. Usually, it was followed by, "Eat it or die." Okay, it wasn't that bad . . . in public.

What I want to stress, here, is that all of this took place at meal time. They didn't burst into my room like the Gestapo and force me to eat avocados while studying for an algebra test. There was no meatball stash under my pillow at night. And, I didn't walk around snacking on pasta noodles all day. Sure, there were snacks, and you had them if you were hungry, but the primary focus was on the three square (or more like, round) meals a day.

> **Food for Thought:**
> *Do I put food in its rightful place, mealtime?*

I'd be remiss if I didn't mention that we always, unless there was an emergency, sat down at the dinner table together, as a family. This was law and, even into the busier high school years, it was expected and demanded. Sure, I resented it a lot at the time, especially in those days.

"Mom, I'm gonna grab a burger with my girlfriend."

"Here. I'm passing the phone to your father. Tell him."

"Hello?"

"Yeah, Dad . . . Uh, just wanted to say, uh, see you at dinner!"

If you were home, you might often hear my mom shout through the house, "Dinner's ready!" or, if it was my dad, "A tavola!" which meant, "To the table!" It was kinda like a battle cry. "A tavola!" "Attack!" And, we'd all storm the table and take no prisoners.

Of course, we never quite got to the table fast enough for my mom. Around supper time, or any time she was cooking for the crew, she had this certain expression on her face. As you got older, you knew what it meant without her having to say a word. Basically, it went like this: "I have slaved for hours in a hot kitchen to put delicious food in your mouths, so you better drop what you're doing right now and get your behind in a seat before I send out my heat-seeking, sauce-tipped, spatula-missile to destroy you."

While she may have been thinking all this, what she said when she had a shred of energy left to say it, was, "'Food's getting cold!" It was amazing. Even if we were having sandwiches for lunch, she would still shout this out through the house.

When I said that food was put in its rightful place, I jokingly followed that with, "our mouths." Yes, that was important, although I admit there were times when I tried the old hide the avocado in the napkin trick or turn over the empty baked potato to serve as a tarp to cover the bitter spinach that I didn't want to eat. Mostly, food went into our mouths, and it happened at the right times, at a pretty regular schedule, morning, noon and night.

And, sure I may have exaggerated about us kids passing out at the table, although I can remember falling asleep as a pipsqueak at restaurants or weddings, sprawled out across two chairs after one too many Shirley Temples and a full, satisfying meal. I think that's the key, though. It was pretty much drilled into me that meal time was when you were satisfied with food. This is very important and I very much appreciate it.

We had fruit after the main course and the occasional dessert, though you were full enough from dinner that you didn't overdo the sweets at the end. So, while I may have stretched a little in saying pasta was at the top of our food pyramid, I do remember all of our meals being balanced well. Mom always managed to have a good source of protein, veggies, and, yes, carbohydrates at supper time. Add in a healthy helping of about three quarts of olive oil per meal and you were good to go!

[20]

So, with all this, you might wonder how I could turn out a chubby kid. I wouldn't say I was obese. I was a little on the chunky side, but this may have been baby fat that was just hanging around . . . until college.

Really, and this is important, too: it was all about self-perception. As a kid growing up in a New York community, I fit right in. We used pizzas as Frisbees, threw stuffed peppers at each other on the dodge ball line. When we moved out West to Scottsdale, Arizona, I felt like Columbus in a New World. Here I was, pale-skinned, strangely accented and a bit portly, among natives (those indigenous to that area) who were thin as rails and tan as rawhide.

So, perception was key. I felt out of place. However, it never occurred to me to eat differently. I really didn't need to. My parents monitored us on sweets. We didn't overdo it. My parents never told me in direct or indirect ways to watch what I ate, or else I'd become a fatso. In fact, it was almost the opposite. They were still stuck in the Renaissance era,

Food for Thought: If you're a parent, what foundation are you laying for your child's relationship with food?

I think. To them, chubby was good. It meant they were doing their job.

As much as I felt different, I still had a good self-esteem built-in from my parents. It wasn't entirely weight-

[21]

based. They taught me to be proud of who I was, and that I didn't have to be like everyone else. Of course, in retrospect, I realize this was also a way to get me to wear polyester hand-me-downs.

Unfortunately, kids today, as a majority, cannot say the same thing (no, not about polyester!). Their parents are generally more preoccupied with weight than their parents before them. This transfers very easily onto children and how they view food and their own bodies.

Over time, with more activity, since I wasn't snowed in half the year in AZ, I shed the weight and, while I never exactly fit in with the locals, I trimmed up a bit. And, really, this was primarily due to the climate change. We went on eating the same way we always had, although the fish wasn't as fresh and the special New York products were few and far between.

For the rest of my childhood, my relationship with food stayed consistent and relatively healthy. So, when did it start to sour? Generally, that depended on the expiration date. No, actually, it got a little rocky, I believe, with the introduction of a little word that had a great deal of impact on me. It's a word that truly holds most of the world's population hostage and hugely affects our diet. I bet you can guess what it is. Turn to the next chapter and let's see!

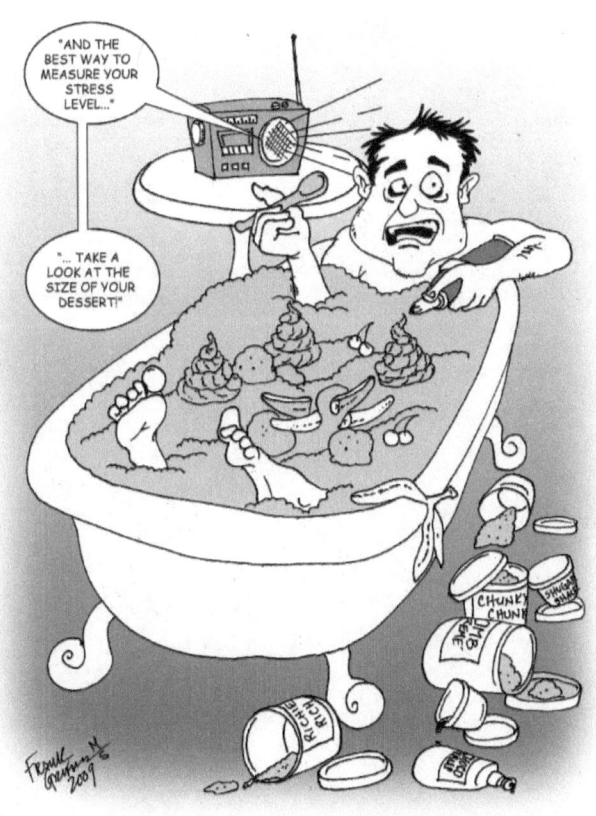

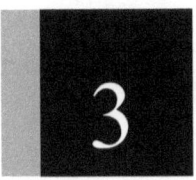

3

Where Did I Go Wrong?
(Why doesn't food call me anymore? I thought we had something special.)

Stress. It's the nasty, little, six-letter word that most of us are quite familiar with. I distinctly remember being introduced to it about the same time I was introduced to another dreaded word: Chemistry. This was the first subject in my schooling career that I couldn't fake my way through and that I just couldn't find any way on earth to connect with. I mean, how often, in your everyday life, do you bring up the Periodic Table?

"Bob, I'd like to schedule a board meeting on Thursday, lunch time."

"Hold on. Let me consult my Periodic Table first. No, sorry. I can't do it then."

"Why not?"

"Don't ask me! I hated Chemistry!"

Looking back, I seem to remember experiencing a good deal of stress in my later high school years, staying up to study for exams, especially in the subjects I hated most. I would be tired and often doubtful if I could cover the material I needed to cover in one night. So, I would make myself a bowl of cereal. It wasn't a bowl of Bran Flakes, mind you, or Shredded Cardboard. There was definitely a sweetness factor involved.

Now, I didn't do this, thinking, "Gosh, I'm really stressed. I think I should feed that stress with something tasty!"

Part of me really thought it would help me stay up longer. Of course, after the sugar high wore off, I'd be a walking zombie. Time to pour another bowl!

You have to understand. This was back in the day before children were regular coffee drinkers. Nowadays, I see children who can't be older than eight or nine, bopping around the local coffee shop.

"How cute! They'll be ordering a hot chocolate," I'm thinking. "Or, a decaf at the most." No, these kids sidle up to the counter and order regular coffee drinks just like the rest of us! Granted, they're mostly disguised as milkshakes, but still! Isn't this alarming to anyone other than me? What are parents thinking? Sure, let's give them sugar *and* caffeine! Add on top of this some *Eminem* lyrics and we've got a community crisis waiting to happen.

No, my mom didn't whip up an espresso to help me through those late study nights. I set myself up with a little treat and so began the long association with late nights, stress and a bowl of sweet cereal. Funny how, years later, during our second year of marriage, when my wife and I had just gotten our little baby girl down to bed, I'd find myself hankering for something sweet. It was probably one of the most stressful years of my life, starting a new job in a new field, in a new state, starting a family, and, wouldn't you know, starting in on a bowl of cereal at least once a night.

Looking back, I could almost hear a variation on that 70's song playing in the background, "Here come the pounds, la, la, la, la. Here come the pounds, and I say, it's all right!"

Um, no. It's not all right. What happened was that I was using food for a purpose other than what it was made for. Almost twelve years later, I've seen a lot.

> *Food for Thought:*
> *How do I handle stress? In a healthy or unhealthy way?*

I've watched my body change with the seasons, with each pregnancy my wife has gone through, each career up or down, and I've come to realize the core problem with me and food.

People say stress is bad. Don't feed the stress. It's not that simple, the way I figure. Stress is always going to be in your life, unless of course, you're dead. There's always going to be something weighing on your mind, some problem you're grappling with, some challenge, some pain deep within.

We don't eat poorly because we're stressed. We eat poorly because that stress makes us unhappy and we think the big piece of chocolate cake is going to reverse that.

Yes, food makes me happy. And, yes, that's my problem.

I came to this realization a while ago, and I think it's the biggest secret to the weight gain problem that nobody wants to talk about.

It's time to ask yourself how your relationship with food is. Go on. Think about it. What are you using it for?

❖ When you're afraid, do you want to run home and hide inside a giant candy bar wrapper (after you've devoured the chocolate inside)?

❖ On the job, or driving to and from work, do you need to suck on a two hundred ounce soda pop like a baby needing to nurse for comfort?

❖ When you're bored, do you find yourself eating recreationally?

❖ Do you have rituals that just can't be altered? You *gotta* have something to munch on during the movie or the game, or the TV show. "Hey, it's nine o'clock. Kids are in bed. This is *my* time, finally . . . to eat."

How embarrassing is this next situation? Once or twice my wife and I have had to tell one of the kids, "No, you can't have ice cream or candy before bed. That's not healthy. Now, goodnight." Then, once we checked the radar and the sonar, and were sure there was no movement or sound upstairs, we popped on a video and broke out the bowls of ice cream to kick back and enjoy . . . only to hear a small voice from the shadows of our staircase ask, "What're you guys eating?"

Have you ever had to respond to this one? You feel like the biggest heel on the planet. Short of lying, "No, this isn't ice cream! It's a frozen vitamin soup—tastes very disgusting," you find yourself scrambling for the only justification you can find. "Well, son, when you're older you can do things like this!" That's great. Really setting a fine example there!

❖ At mealtimes, have you found yourself going back for a second or third helping only because it tasted good? "I know I shouldn't, but I think I'll have myself four more scoops of those garlic mashed potatoes."

Again, we don't see this in third world countries. You don't hear someone in Ethiopia say, "That bean curd was so good, I think I'll load up my plate again and wipe out next week's supply."

❖ Have you become a sweets junkie, where you're always looking for the next good fix? "You know, that bag of Oreos was good, but it just didn't quite hit the spot! Let's try chocolate chip!"

❖ How about the infamous salty-sweet-salty-sweet cycle? Ever found yourself in this one? "Those pretzels were salty! Now I need something sweet!" Minutes later, "Whew, that candy was sweet. I could use something salty . . ." And the cycle continues . . . until you pass out.

❖ When you're stressed, depressed, having a bad day, do you turn to food for solace? The thing about depression is—and I know this because I've been there—the food doesn't even taste good to you, but you keep eating it, hoping it will kick in at some point. There should be a bumper sticker or T-shirt made up that says, "Life's tough. Eat hard." This is what we do, isn't it?

> **Food for Thought:**
> *Am I addicted to food?*

❖ Has food become the one and only thing you can depend on in this world to always be there for you, to give you that rush of enjoyment and satisfaction that you long for?

And here, really, lies the crux of the whole situation. Food has become, for a lot of people, the next legal drug. Let's face it, life *is* tough. We have problems, personally. We have situations that are out of our control, and out of control. We have pain that seems unbearable. Are we turning to food just like some people turn to alcohol, sex, gambling, or drugs to make it all better?

When I say food makes me happy and that's my problem, I have to clarify. I'm not stating a literal fact. I'm stating a mindset. I've been *trying* to use food to make me happy. Are you?

EARLY RENAISSANCE SUPER-MODEL ENVY

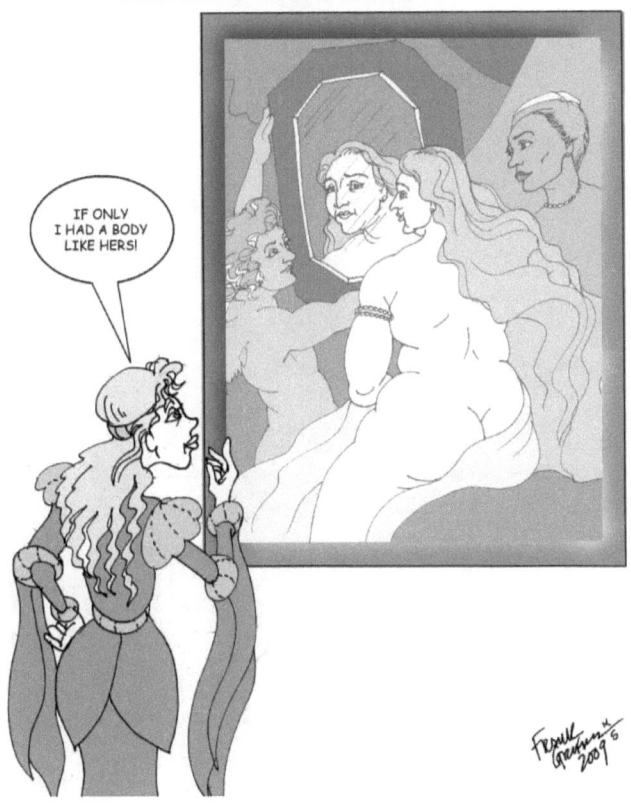

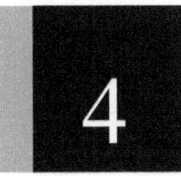

Food Does Not Make Me Happy
(Time to face the music)

Just like any other drug or addiction, there's always the promise, beforehand, of fulfillment, of satisfaction. Do you get this violently strong feeling sometimes? For example, when someone offers dessert after a meal, do your legs start shaking, palms get a little sweaty? Do you find your pulse quickening a little as you walk through the frozen treats aisle at the grocery store?

Is there an adrenaline rush as you dig through the ice cream shelf like an Eskimo hunter, searching for that special flavor? You suffer frost-bite. Maybe you're even willing to lose a finger in order to find the right one, the cherished one. At last, you tear off the lid and there it is, that perfect, unblemished surface of silky pleasure. You dig right in. Hopefully, this isn't on the way to the check-out counter. Hopefully, you haven't locked yourself in the freezer to guard the remaining few gallons of your precious treasure as you eat through them all right then and there, afraid someone might cart-jack you on the way to the cashier.

Fast-forward five, ten, minutes. Maybe thirty, depending on how well you can "put 'em down." The high begins to fade. That feeling of, "I never thought something could taste so darn good in all my ever-loving life" starts to change into something else.

Here, we enter the let-down phase: "Um, you know, that triple layer fudge brownie ice cream with mint chips, caramel waves, toffee shell and cookie core didn't really taste as good as I remembered."

There's also the guilt. You're at someone's house and you find yourself confiding in them, even if you don't know them that well. "Why did I do that? I shouldn't have had that last piece of pie."

"You had the last half of the pie."

"Okay, it was a big piece! What's wrong with me?!"

There's the sick feeling. "I can't move. Someone's going to have to carry me from the table to the couch. Careful when you lift me, boys! My belt's unbuckled! Easy! Easy!"

"No, not so easy, bub!"

Or, have you ever found yourself saying this one after you've overindulged? "I feel like I'm going to throw up, I ate so much!" Hmmm. Sound like any Romans you used to know?

The raw truth of the matter is that food does not a happy person make. It gives nourishment and, when used properly, it sustains life, working together with other factors to make a whole and complete person. When it is abused, however, it can make you sick. Certainly, it can make you feel gross at the time, but its misuse can also cause serious health problems: obesity, diabetes, heart problems, vision problems, high blood pressure, eating disorders . . . and these are just the ones you hear about.

These things are undeniable, scientifically speaking, and most people know them. Why can't we stop, though? If we know our car is low on brake fluid, we don't generally take a pleasure trip through the mountains at speeds up to 90 mph, do we? No, we know better. We exercise some control there.

So, why is it so hard to get a grip on the food situation? I think the answer is that it is not merely a physical, mechanical, cause and effect relationship. Food is entwined with our emotional and mental state to such a degree that it becomes not just one aspect of our life, but a main focus. Whether we realize it or not, we are obsessed with it. It has a strong hold on us that we're usually not aware of.

Let's take a look at a case study. I'm not a doctor or a psychologist, so I can't refer to a patient. I will, however, refer to someone I know very well. In fact, I'll combine

[35]

myself along with people I know and/or have observed in my life and I'll make an amalgam. Since I don't want to name any names or even do the acronym thing (because, no doubt some genius will figure out who I'm talking about), I'll give this example a fictitious name: Fatty Johnson.

Okay, that's not very nice. Let's try a more common name: Baluga. No, um, that's the name of a whale. Sorry, I'm really bad with names. Let's use one that's not gender specific, too. How about Sam? There you go—could go either way.

Now, Sam worked at a very stressful job. Sam, being a great manager, brought donuts in every morning to improve office morale. Sam usually ended up eating all of them throughout the day, even the plain one without chocolate or anything on it, because Sam felt sorry for it being left in the box all by itself. Sam thought about Sam's meals a lot. Before Sam was barely finished with breakfast, Sam was wondering what the meal for lunch would be.

Sam needed a snack before lunch and did not feel guilty about this, since no human being could be expected to last four hours without eating something. Thus, a coffee and three Danishes were generally well justified. Sam tried to be sensible with lunch. Just a salad and maybe a bag of chips with a diet cola. Problem was, Sam craved something sweet after lunch. It distracted Sam to no end. Sam couldn't move on with life or work or even bare existence without satisfying that craving. Chocolate was needed, for the good of Sam, for the good of Sam's work and personal circle, as well.

Sam would find sweet relief and then, after struggling to stay awake the rest of the afternoon, Sam would suffer through until dinner. This was feast time that served as a reward for the day's work, with large portions that stretched the limits of Sam's already overstretched stomach. However, oddly enough, only an hour or two after dinner, Sam was hungry again. Maybe Sam was reading. Most likely, Sam was couched in front of the TV watching an unending offering of favorite shows. Naturally, for stamina and even company, Sam had a bag of chips and/or a bowl or two of ice cream along for the ride.

> **Food for Thought:**
> *Am I Sam? (or, for all of you Dr. Seuss fans – Sam I am?)*

Sam would fall asleep on the couch if Sam couldn't break through the fog and stumble into bed before collapsing. Strange dreams and frequent trips to the bathroom dotted Sam's night due to eating so late, and so, sluggishly and somewhat disgruntled, Sam would awake the next day to start the process all over again.

Now this isn't to say that Sam didn't get anything accomplished at work or maintain a relationship or two. That's the great deception, here. Food is the quiet controller. You don't realize it has a hold of you until one morning you look in the mirror and you're twice the person you used to be.

I've often wondered what would happen if today's societal perceptions changed back to those of the Renaissance times, when fullness was fashion. Would the issues with food simply fade away or not? Is it really all the media's fault? Is it really just a matter of self-perception and comparison?

Food for Thought:
How do I feel about myself when I see supermodels?

You can't go into a grocery store nowadays without seeing a dozen or so magazine covers of human sculptures seemingly carved with an artist's knife (or airbrush) to perfection. They're all smiling and happy, successful and strong. Consciously or subconsciously, we compare ourselves, and the message is clear: you can't be happy unless you look like those people on the covers.

Was it this way, post-Middle Ages? Did someone walk through the Sistine Chapel and think, "Man, if only I was as plump as those people in the frescoes, then my life would really turn around!" Well, on some level, I'm sure it was. Usually, if you were that full-figured, it meant you could afford a decent meal or three per day, and this was always good. It's funny how looking well-fed was a positive reflection back then, and, today, looking starved or barely nourished is "in."

Turn on the TV and it's inhabited by skinny, fashionable people. Unless, of course, your show is a satirical, sad look at how a fat person tries to fit in or lose weight. Why do most, if not all commercials feature thin people to sell the products?

There's no denying that, straight up from grade school there's a new class warfare in this country, between those who are the "hottest" and those who don't come close. Why do kids pick on their chubbier classmates? Do their parents send them off to school with a clear directive on this?

"Okay, now, son. Have a nice day. And, remember, if you see someone who's on the plump side, be sure to mock them without mercy."

That's absurd! But, why is it that even children know about weight distinction? Sure, it's the media they're exposed to. If all they ever see as normal and happy is the trim person, they don't know any better. And, yes, parents play a role. Their attitudes rub off on their children in ways they never imagined.

I remember when my son was around seven, one day he was excitedly telling me about a candy bar he'd eaten earlier. "And it had 300 calories!" was the last in a list of feverish, gooey descriptions.

I was really careful in my reply, because, first of all, how on earth does my little son know to count calories?! Never mind that, he's picked it up from us. Nothing to do now except set his mind straight and lay the foundation of a good attitude toward food.

"Son," I said. "First of all, that's a big candy bar! Second of all, you should be ashamed of yourself!"

No, I didn't say that. In reality, I was just excited for him. And, as he talked on, he told me how he split the large chocolate bar with a friend, since, in his words, "I know too much sweets aren't good for you!"

Of course, I told him he was right, and I smiled to myself, hoping this level-headed attitude of his would last.

The other reason I think some kids pick on the heavier child in class is because they want to make themselves look and feel better. Sure, this isn't a ground-breaking thought, but it's important to note. Maybe it's just my kids, but I haven't "seen" any of the four of them show any tendency toward discriminating against anyone for any reason. We've tried hard to instill an all-encompassing, "love thy neighbor" mentality in them.

I believe kids start out this way. Then, when you throw them into a socially competitive environment, suddenly, whether they realize it or not, they are vying for position and power, and suddenly (not my kids, of course!) they're putting someone down to make themselves look better.

The reason I bring this up is for us to be aware, as I'm sure we've all seen, that an attitude like this can continue on all through middle school, high school, college, and even clear into old age for some people. They are so insecure with themselves that these people must find a way to feel better, even at the expense of others. And, whose expense is it all too often? The person who doesn't fit the social norm (as dictated by media and fashion trends, and conditioned into our minds). They are the easy target.

> **Food for Thought:** *Do I see people around me as my competition or as companions along the way of life?*

Nothing new here. But, here's a point you may not have considered before: Many people, including myself at times, are both the bully <u>and</u> the victim. I don't mean in separate instances, though that happens, too. I mean, at the same time. *We pick on ourselves.* We make fun of ourselves. God forbid, but we even HATE ourselves.

How can this be, you ask? Well, no one ever said a man's best friend is himself. And no one would even dare suggest it about a woman. It saddens me to no end how women especially tend to despise themselves because they don't look the way they think they should.

Here it is, again. We all want to fit in and feel like we belong. Intentionally or not, the media powers have created an "in" group. You look like this and act like this or you don't belong.

Don't belong where, you ask? I mean, for adults, we're not at school anymore, so . . . yeah, well, there's work, and that's as bad as grade school sometimes, certainly, but I'm talking about *life*! Some people believe they don't belong in life itself because they don't fit in to the norms of society!

This is heartbreaking. They believe that, everywhere they go, the grocery store, the bank, walking down the street, they are being judged. Somewhere, someone is thinking to themselves, "Wow, that person is really disgusting! What's wrong with them?"

Now, there may not be an actual person standing there doing that. If there is, all I have to say to that person is, "What's wrong with you?! Take a look inside yourself and spend the rest of your life working on *that,* why don't you!?" Sorry, but I'm taking the gloves off now. Look out!

Regardless of whether the person is there or not, the comment is said or not, the side-long glance or the snobbish dismissal has occurred, the self-loathing person still feels the way he or she does. It's conditioning of the worst kind. (Don't worry, we're going to discuss ways of rinsing it out a little later, you can bet!)

Food, in these cases, becomes the enemy. But, it's an enemy that's easy to love. Yes, we've entered into that old love-hate relationship, here. A self-deprecating person, stuck in the dreadful mind-trap of societal norms, will curse food for making them so miserable. But then, since they are so miserable, they can't help but run back into the arms of food to relieve their pain. Remember, it's the next legal drug, after all.

People who are obsessed with their weight or body figure (and believe me, I've been there at times) often find themselves looking at the fit jogger or the nearly transparent woman ordering the latte and wishing upon every star that they were them. Yes, like their Renaissance counterpart, they're in the great, neighborhood Coffee Chapel and they're fantasizing about how much better their life would be if only they had the perfect body.

It's my firm opinion though, that the coffee isn't always blacker on the other side . . .

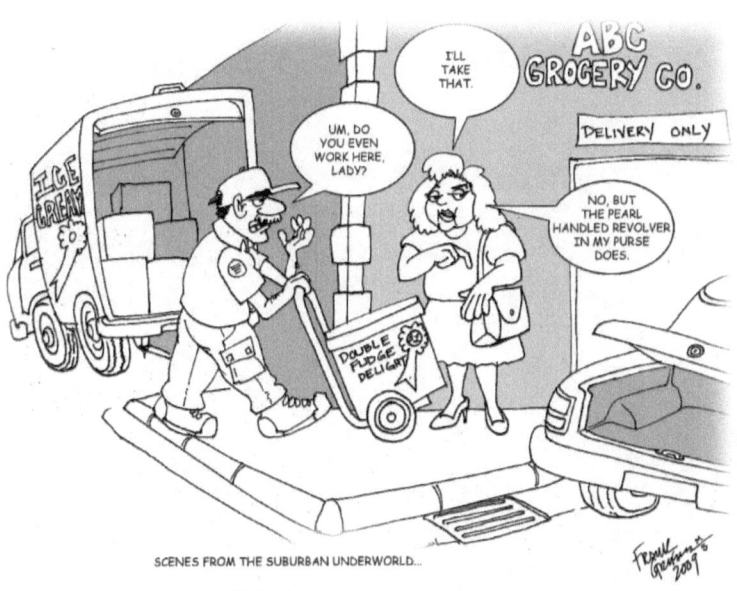

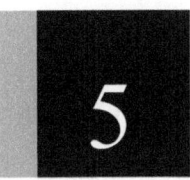

My Body Doesn't Make Me Happy Either
(Really.)

Warning: This chapter may upset, confuse or downright anger some of you. You're just going to have to trust me, okay? And, if you're an advertising executive, you may just want to put the book down now and walk away.

Here's the deal. I might as well just come out and say it: Primarily focusing on looking good and feeling good is not going to make you happy.

Yes, you read that right. Having the perfect body, as much as everything in print, celluloid and such wants to convince you otherwise, does not equal having the perfect life.

We're not dealing with the law of opposites here. Just because Donny is sad all the time because he's overweight, doesn't mean that making him underweight will make him totally happy, either.

"Now, stop right there," you might say. "I know plenty of people who say their lives have improved dramatically since they lost a lot of weight!"

"Really?" would be my reply. "Their lives improved *dramatically*, huh? What did they tell you?"

Then, you'd come back at me with a barrage of common post-pound-reduction comments that float around public and private circles. What I'm going to do now is scientifically dissect these statements and prove to you just how deceiving they can be.

Comment #1: "Oh, I've never felt so good!"

My Answer: Really? What about those midnight cravings for chocolate cake that send you climbing up the walls, huh?! Oh, the depravation! And the constant counting of calories and the paranoia that someday, when you least expect it, the weight will return?

Comment #2: "I can fit into all of my old clothes again!"

My Answer: Who says we want to see you in those old rags again?

Comment #3: "I'm making more friends than ever before!"

My Answer: If they are only attracted to you when you're "attractive," are these really the kind of friends you want?

Okay, now, I know those responses may be a little extreme. Sure, it's good to feel good about yourself, to wear those clothes you never thought you could, and to gain the confidence to meet new people. My point

> **Food for Thought:**
> *Do I gauge my happiness for the day based on how I look in the mirror or on how I feel inside?*

is that, just like the pleasure of eating food is a momentary thing, passing as quickly as sugar is absorbed into your bloodstream, so is the happiness gained by superficial, exterior looks.

So, this begs the question: Why do you want to lose weight? Is it so you can say all of the above comments and more? Is it because you think you can't be happy until you look just right?

Here is yet another subtle truth that no one, especially the "diet" people and facial cream people, want you to know: YOU ARE GOING TO BECOME UGLY. Try as you might, you can't fight aging; you can't fight gravity. Your nose will never stop growing, or your ear lobes, until the day you die. Sunspots, varicose veins, corns, strange growths, excessive nose, ear and back hair . . . yes, they're on their way, too!

Don't get me wrong. By "ugly," I mean according to society's standards. Why do you think the elderly have become so generally despised and dispensable? They're just not fitting the mold. They're cramping our style. Never mind that they are a storehouse of wisdom, tradition, experience and love, not to mention opportunities for us to serve and grow as selfless caregivers. That's not the beauty *we're* interested in! (I hope you sense the sarcasm here.)

And, that's the big question: What kind of beauty are you interested in?

If the answer is bodily beauty, then I want you to do the following exercise. Please, really do this. Go out and buy yourself a big bag of cotton candy. Pink, purple, red, blue, whatever color suits your fancy. If you can't find it at the grocery store, go to an amusement park or the state fair. It'll be worth the trip.

Now, then. Rip off a big chunk of that cloud-like, edible fly-trap material and shove it in your mouth. Now, pay careful attention here, because, before you can even think about chewing, it's gone! It's dissolved down to nothing, with just the hint and memory of sugar left (along with the ripe promise of tooth decay!).

I'm just telling you, if you're building your foundation of happiness on how you look, you're trying to live off cotton candy.

Let's do this. We'll take Bob as our next example. Bob's a bit bubbly in the waistline. Okay, he's a size 40 inseam. Bob's depressed. He wishes he were slender like those guys in the infomercials. He actually orders one of their ab-contraptions, the one on wheels, but after rolling down the stairs and nearly dying during a strenuous work-out session, Bob gets his money back. Next, he decides to get a personal trainer. The people at the gym scare him, so he swallows his pride and asks his next door neighbor, a sports doctor, to help him out. The man gives him some pointers and Bob's on his way.

Trouble is, Bob combines his new medical pointers with the "advice" from a popular teen magazine that suggests starvation and lots of running (great combo). Bob becomes obsessed. He's not the Bob his family or co-workers used to know. He runs all the time, barely eats, but is deliriously happy to see the weight falling off. Two months later, Bob is at his desired weight. He's built a little muscle, too and, while he's no infomercial star yet, Bob starts to feel really good about Bob.

Yes, life is just grand for Bob now. He climbs out of the shower and is no longer ashamed to look at himself in the mirror. In fact, if he could, he would grace the neighborhood with his nakedness, just to show everyone how happy he is with himself. Something goes wrong for Bob, as you might expect. No, he's not arrested for indecent exposure!

His car battery needs changing. He goes to the mechanic's and, during a routine inspection, yep, you guessed it, Bob is sprayed in the face with acid. The damage is permanent and, as we all know from The Phantom of the Opera, masks will just never be "in." Where does all Bob's happiness go now? Remember the cotton candy?

Okay, this is an extreme example, you say? Consider Cindy, then. She jogs at least two hours a day, one in the morning, one at night. She's always obsessing over her weight. In fact, she's become a walking calorie counter and, if she goes a little over, like maybe accidentally eating a crouton in her salad, she makes herself pay for it with an extra hour at the gym that night.

Yes, Cindy likes how men admire her from a distance, like she's some sort of goddess of beauty. She likes how the kid at the coffee counter stumbles over his words, and someone usually burns their hands on the espresso machine because they're so caught up in awe of her.

Now, because an object of beauty is in great danger of being objectified, Cindy has a rough time with intimate relationships. In the past, she's mistaken the charm of men who just want a shot at being in her deific presence (and bedroom), for sincere appreciation. Maybe she, too, has begun to value others on superficial, outside qualities. Could she ever see herself dating a short, dumpy guy? What if her own preoccupation with external beauty has blinded her from seeing where true love really lies? Due to all this and past disappointments, her only source of solace come from that which she feels she can control: her physical appearance.

What happens to Cindy, then, over time? What if she gets sick, therefore missing her morning jogs and daily trips to the gym? What if she has a baby? Will she resent the child for the weight it brings her? Will she avoid having children for this reason, and thereby miss out on all of the joy that comes from motherhood? Regardless of the answers to these questions, the one, undeniable fact is that Cindy will, like the rest of us, grow old. Her body will do things she does not want it to do. Is she ready to accept this?

> **Food for Thought:** *Am I ready to accept that I'm getting older every day?*

At the writing of this book, I'm 35. Asking myself this question, I find a mixed answer, if I want to be honest about it. No, I'm not ready to accept it. I still want to see myself as the young guy I used to be. Grey hair? That's for my dad, not me! And, shoulder hair! What's that about? No one ever told me about shoulder hair. No, I don't have carpet-like patches of hair on my shoulders, but I've got a nice collection of strays that are just as perplexing and disturbing. They make it look like I have two balding heads as book-ends of my upper torso. Ask anyone in my family and they'll tell you (not with great pride, mind you) how

I've affectionately dubbed my shoulders Uncle Louie and Uncle Herman.

So, yes, I have a sense of humor about it.

I just told my wife the other night that she will someday have to knit a separate sweater for me for my nose. Yes, it's a big, Roman nose now. But, look out, people, it's still on the move! That puppy's not going to stop growing until my heart stops. If I make it to old age, it's going to be quite a honker, I must say!

So, how does this make me feel? Sure, sometimes it's tough to reconcile. The problem is a two-fold one with me. First, and I know I'll get into trouble on this one, I would have to cite my wife. Now, I need to be careful here (not out of fear, no, but love and respect) so I'll start by saying, she's a good person, a great person! Like other wives, however, she sometimes gets caught up in the outward, physical appearance of her husband in a slightly unhealthy fashion. Maybe it's because she wants us to fight aging together or still feel like we can match that youthful honeymoon picture, but, occasionally she'll let slip a comment or two about my looks that will send me reeling just like an insecure teenager again.

I'm not talking about general hygiene or appearance upkeep remarks, like, "Hey, thought about showering after working in the yard, before jumping into bed?" or "Hi, these are nail clippers. I'd like to formally introduce them to you."

[54]

No, I'm referring to the subtle, "Hmm, 'lot of grey up there," or "Huh, I wonder what those shoulders would be like without curly hair?" or "Pants a little tight, there, chubby—I mean, hubby!?"

Like I said, she's a very decent human being. I'm sure she doesn't even realize what she's saying at the time. I know she's been conditioned to evaluate and pass judgment on a superficial level. I have been. We all have!

That's the second part of my problem: self-perception. Yes, imagine that. I'm still struggling with how I look at myself and judge my appearance. Why do I still hold my gut in when I look sideways in a mirror? Do you see how ingrained and deviously transparent the lie has become? A person such as me can talk about and firmly believe in placing value on myself and others by the truth of who they are as opposed to what they look like, while still, on a near daily basis, face the mirror and suck it in.

It's amazing how much widespread preoccupation there is with one's appearance. We've discussed earlier how all of us have this desire to fit in and belong, and how the media has set up the definitions for "the place" to be at, and "the mold" to fit, however, we can't let the blame stop there. We have ourselves to blame.

"Yes, I've been brainwashed! Oh, poor me! I'm a victim of the system!"

No, that's not gonna fly, either. I am responsible for my thoughts, my attitudes and my actions at any and every given moment. I have to, first of all, be aware that I'm buying into the lie that my body will make me happy, and then I have to forcibly remove the hook from my mouth, regardless of the pain.

Yes, I know that the advertising executive who did not heed my warning and is still reading this chapter, has now got his/her hand on the phone receiver about to order a contract out on my life, but, fearlessly, I must go on!

It's time, my friends, to reverse the conditioning that we've undergone, to rinse it out forcibly and with uncommon vigor! Oh, yes, it's slick! It's been applied in gross amounts for many, many years, and it's really more like petroleum jelly than hair softener, so look out! This will not be easy. It will not happen overnight. But, I promise you, it will happen and it will be worth it.

It is a subject that really could take volumes to dissect and discuss, and more worthy and scholarly people than myself have probably done just that. However, it's a key element in the progression toward a healthy relationship with food, and so I must take a moment to lay out my plan for this. At the risk of being overly simplistic, I've outlined two-- count them, two-- easy steps to breaking the superficial, physical-appearance mindset.

Here they are:

Step 1:
Believe that any real value worth mentioning comes not from what you look like, but who you are.

You've believed the opposite for so long, why not try the truth on for a change? I could use the example of Mother Theresa, here-- a truly amazing spirit contained within a hunched, tiny, wrinkled form-- but it would be a bad example. This might give the impression that what you do outwardly equates to what you're worth. Sure, it's important to do good for others, but, when you truly look at yourself, you must start with the beautiful, core reality shared by belief systems across the globe, that all human beings are equally precious and valuable, no matter what their age, shape, color, size, accomplishments, creed, or any other distinguishing attribute.

Step 2:

You can't just say, "Yes, I believe that now." You have to, on a daily, if not moment by moment basis, remind yourself of this simple, freeing truth.

Food for Thought: How many attractive people do you see out there doing the work of Mother Theresa?

You have to live it, breathe it in, and use it to break free of the chains of negative self-perception! When you find yourself sizing up someone else based on their physical appearance, you need to literally remind yourself, "This is a human being, precious and equal to me and everyone else." The same rule applies to yourself.

[57]

Here we go. Take this book, now. Go into your bathroom, not the public one, because, what I'm going to ask you to do might get you arrested . . . if not done in private. Okay. Are you there, yet? No? I'll wait. I've got time.

Alright, once you've locked the door and you're facing a mirror, I want you to strip down. Yes, you read right. No, I'm not a perverted person. The human body is a beautiful work of art in all of its stages, with all of its perfections and imperfections. You don't have to get all naked, here. Just reveal some flesh, preferably in the areas that you are most self-conscious about. For me, it would be my belly and, yes, my hairy shoulders. Thanks for reminding me.

Now, I want you to start first with your eyelashes. Most of us still have these. Get up close to the mirror and examine those tiny, identical strands of hair that come out of the ends of your eyelids. Run your finger gently across them. Aren't they amazing? So neatly lined up, so firm in their shape to protect your eye from pollen, dust and kamikaze gnats! And, if one falls out, what happens? Another one just like it grows back in its place! You don't have to call the eyelash manufacturer and place an order. You don't have to find your owner's manual and figure out the right way to replace the one you lost. It just works! It pops out without you giving it a second thought. It's truly amazing.

[58]

Look into your eyes now. Look deep and true and clear. If you're uncomfortable with this, get over it. I mean, come on. It's you! You should be used to yourself by now! A famous saying is that the eyes are a window to a person's soul. Before you get that deep, I want you to just marvel at how your eyeball works. Pretty crazy, huh? Catching the light, breaking it down into an image your brain can process. Note, if you've lost an eye, or you are blind, don't take this to mean that you are any less than the person who hasn't or isn't. Move on to your nose. That's an amazing fixture, isn't it?

I think you can get the picture of what I'm telling you to do, here. I want you to marvel at your fundamental, human beauty. Marvel at how your body knows to send white blood cells to a cut you get on your finger and, without you even thinking about it, works daily to heal that wound until there's barely a trace of it left. Look at your fingerprint. Remember how mind-boggling it is that there's no other like it, nor has there ever been or will be in this world! Look at those thumbs. Kiss those thumbs! They allow you to do so much! After all, where would The Fonze be without them?

Take time with this. Go over everything. All of you is precious and amazing, not because it fits some societal mold, but because it is *you*! It is inseparably part of who you are and, therefore, it only follows that, if you are unspeakably valuable, so is every part and sum total of your body.

[59]

Hold it. We're not done here. I know some of you, just like me, quickly breezed by those areas of our body that we find less than satisfactory or downright disgusting. Don't walk away from that thought. Let's analyze it.

Is it a patch of cellulite? Is it sagging skin that you wish you could have tucked, or a misplaced mole? Is it a part of you that you wish was bigger, smaller, different? The important question you need to ask yourself, right now, as you're staring it down, is why? Why, really? If you could snap your fingers and have it magically change to the way you wanted it to be, would you be happy? If you answered yes, go to the start of this chapter and start reading again.

Why is that part of you, or even the

Please remember this key phrase: "My value is not based on how I look."

whole sum of you something you perceive as bad or in need of improvement? Is it because you are placing it up alongside some supermodel, movie star, co-worker, or infomercial star you have stored in your mind that you will forever compare yourself against? Stop! From this moment on, see yourself for <u>who</u> you are and, dare I say it, love yourself for exactly that. Love yourself, value yourself for the pure and simple fact that you are you, and you are entirely and utterly irreplaceable, no matter what anyone tells you or makes you feel, including yourself! You may or may not fit the societal norm for beauty at this stage in your life. Who the hell cares!? Look at yourself. Don't worry about anybody else or what anyone else looks like or thinks of you. (Remember, I'm telling myself to do this, too, because God knows I need to at times!) Tell yourself, I don't have to look like a supermodel to have value.

Repeat with me: "My value is not based on how I look. My value is not based on how I look. My value is not based on how I look. Hmm. What should I have for dinner tonight?" Whoah! See how that sneaks in there?! See how easy it is to get distracted and pulled away from the truth?

For those with eating disorders, or if you know of anyone who feels they need to either starve themselves or make themselves throw up after eating, this is especially crucial. We need to make sure these people get help. And, that they don't feel ashamed about it. We all need help for different things, at different times.

This is urgent, however. It's a serious illness that can lead to major health complications and death. It's been documented over and over, and I've seen it, sadly, in the circles of friends and acquaintances in my lifetime. Depriving yourself of the recommended calories and nutrition for your specific age and make-up is deadly.

If you're in this boat, know that you're not alone, that everyone struggles with self image. You're hurting right now, you're sick. But, it can be turned around. The foundation starts with loving yourself again (Yes, there was a time when you did, when we all did. As very young children, we didn't give a second thought to how we looked. We were who we were, and we were at peace with it without even thinking about it. We all need to go back to that.) .

And, please don't think that reading the above few paragraphs is going to instantly solve the problem. If you have an eating disorder, you need to confide in someone close to you and have them help you get counseling. Again, nothing to be ashamed of. If all of us were truly honest with ourselves, we'd all be in counseling for one reason or another. We all need to strive to be healthier. If you have an eating disorder, your situation is life and death, so it must be addressed *now*. There are plenty of agencies out there to help. At the writing of this book, a place to find help and resources is the National Eating Disorders Association's 24-hour information and referral toll-free helpline: 1-800-931-2237.

Okay, back to the mirror. There you are in all your glory. Yes, I mean that. Now, you might be thinking, "I don't want to look like the next supermodel. I just want to be healthy and look healthy."

Fine. I'll give you that. But, will you not be happy with yourself, at peace with yourself, or love yourself until you reach that point? And, what if you do, but then your health declines? People always say that the most important thing is that you have your health. Um, hello? What happens if that goes bye-bye? Ask anyone struck by cancer or any other debilitating disease out of the blue. This is a major blow, to say the least. So, it only follows that you can't base your happiness on your health, either.

Now, I'm not saying it doesn't matter if you're healthy, or, because it doesn't matter how you look, to go ahead and eat like there's no tomorrow. We strive for good health. We do our best to eat right, to exercise, to sleep well, to enrich our minds and souls, and to do all the things necessary to maintain true, good health.

But, at the end of the day, and I hope you can feel the conditioning rinsing clean right at this point, you must look inside yourself and be able to firmly believe that you are who you are meant to be right now. Some of us may have a long way to go to reach healthy. This will require a lot of patience. Some of us are on the teeter totter, back and forth, desiring stability. Some may be at their peak, but are wise enough to know this will not always be the case.

At whatever point we're at, we need to be able to say, "I am a work in progress." Not just any work, priceless artwork. I will be, until the day I die. No one is better than me or less than me. We all have an equal place on the stage of life. Will we dance? Will we sing? Will we spout out a soliloquy with great fervor? Will we play our part to the

[63]

fullest, or will we shrink into the shadows of the wings, saying we're not ready or not good enough to really live?

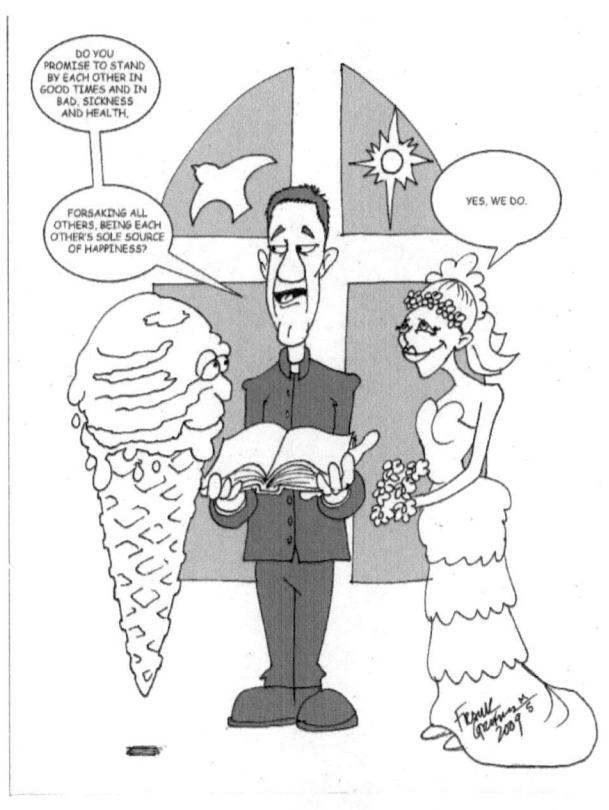

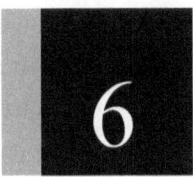

6

What Will Truly Make Me Happy?
(Yes, we can figure it out in only one chapter, trust me!)

Here's the good ole' fashioned toughie of a question: If not based on physical appearance or health, where does happiness lie? I could take the modern, relativist position and say, "It's different for everyone! So, go out and find it, and once you do, you'll be happy!"

Thanks a lot! Big help, there.

Sure, happiness manifests itself in different ways for everyone, but, at least, from what I've learned, it has fundamental principles that will be the same for everyone across the board. Mind you, we're talking about true happiness. I don't mean the kind that lasts one night and you wake up the next morning with a headache and/or various other medical conditions; and I'm not talking about something you buy at the store or dealership, or online.

The two steps you and I took in the previous chapter to break the cycle and see ourselves for who we truly are, i.e., precious and valuable, are great steps. But, how do you live that out?

It's a fundamental desire for us all to want to be happy. But, let's face it. We can't go around all day, thinking to ourselves, "I'm special. I'm special. I'm special," and expect this to be some sort of shield against trials and sorrow. Whether we realize it or not, most of us go about our day trying to figure out ways to make ourselves happy, secure, feel good, fulfilled, etc.

The main focus of this book is how we've fallen into the trap of trying to let food do this for us. "Hey, the bakery never shuts down! There will always be enough cakes and pastries to make *me* happy!"

We know that's not going to cut it, now, but we've also realized something about ourselves. We're not simply creatures of theory. We're physical beings living in a physical world, and we have physical things to deal with: the bullying boss, the angry spouse, the sick child, a chronic case of indigestion, a pestering hangnail, whatever it may be.

So, if we've been in the habit of running to food for comfort, where do we turn to now? A blankie or a favorite pillow? A special person in our lives?

"Yes, that's got to be it! *They* can make me happy. *True love* makes us happy!"

Wrong. People are people, after all. They're not perfect and can't be relied on to make us fulfilled. Of course, they can be part of the picture of happiness, but to say that they are the sole source of happiness, this is a burden no human being can bear. And, it's a dangerous position to put yourself in.

The big irony here is that, while the need for happiness feels very physical, the answer is, dare I say it, spiritual.

"Oh boy," you're thinking. "Here he goes. He's led us down this path to start preaching at us or to push his particular brand of spirituality on us."

Now, don't panic. While I do have a very specific religious inclination and source of spiritual guidance and sustenance in my life (no, it doesn't involve compounds and flavored drink), my goal here is not to enlighten you on that. What I'd like to discuss and help you to understand is a very basic and yes, you guessed it, simple foundation for finding true happiness in life.

I call it spiritual, because we've already ruled out the physical. Remember the cotton candy? We've ruled out our own looks or health being a reliable source for happiness. We've touched on how we can't demand 24/7 fulfillment from another person, i.e., the emotional state.

> **Food for Thought:** *Am I expecting someone in my life to be my source of happiness?*

But, let's stop here for a moment. What about our emotions? After all, isn't happiness a feeling, an emotion? There needs to be a distinction made here. I hate to go all basic and, believe me, I'm not trying to be condescending; I'm just laying a foundation for the argument.

So, is the feeling of happiness the same as real happiness? When a loved one gives you a kiss, or when you score a point, or laugh during a movie, you feel happy, right? Does that mean you *are* happy? Some of you may want to punch me right now. You may want to say, "Happiness is not having to read these annoying questions anymore!"

I know this is unusual and difficult stuff to face, but it's worth working through. Happiness, the emotion, is fleeting. The loved one can certainly slap you moments after kissing you. You can get a tooth knocked out right after scoring. The theater could burn down following a funny part in the flick. Where would that feeling of happiness go, then?

So, you probably felt happy at the time, granted, but the question is, in what state are you living? Happiness, or joy, which is a better term for it, must be a state of being. It's not natural to <u>feel</u> happy all the time. There are times when you need to feel afraid, sad, angry, or otherwise. If someone grabs your wallet, you don't smile and laugh. You get angry, desire justice and dress up like Batman and hunt the thief down.

Okay, maybe you don't go that far. But, let's say you did, and let's carry the situation further. What if you don't find that person? What if you don't get your money back and, suddenly, your credit information is sold to a thousand identity thieves and it's a total nightmare? You're not going to be a happy puppy, are you?

Food for Thought: What state of being do I live in? Joyful? Jaded? Angry, self-pitying, dissatisfied or resentful?

The reaction of anger and sadness over being wronged is a good thing. However, if you add this to the list of why your life is miserable and why you choose to remain in bed for the three weeks reading Henry James novels backwards while gorging on bonbons, then you really need to evaluate your state of being.

If you have joy in your heart, even the toughest trial and most painful emotion cannot root it out.

The next logical thought is what the heck does this guy (meaning me) know about suffering? My answer: Hi, married for nearly fourteen years with four children. What have you got? Not to say that it's all suffering but, hey, there are lows and highs, buddy. Lows and highs.

For the sake of tying back to the title and thread of this book, I'll refer to this unshakeable joy as true happiness. So, where can it be found? If not in a twenty pound cheesecake, then where, for Pete's sake!?

(To be read in a whisper voice) Just so you know, I'm donning a bullet proof vest now as I write this, because the ad execs are really not going to like my next statement. Quick glance out the window. Scanning the nearby rooftops. Looks clear.

Okay, it is my conclusion that <u>the key to finding true happiness for yourself is to stop looking for true happiness for yourself</u>.

Ironic, huh?

To put it simply, self-centeredness equals sadness. Selflessness leads to true happiness. "Hey, wait a minute," you say. "You backed me into a corner, here. You told me we all go about our day looking for ways to make ourselves happy, that this is a pretty common denominator, so now you're saying that it's wrong, that, if I simply stop doing that, I'll be happy?"

My response to those valid questions, thank you, is, first of all, look at the world as we know it. Would you say that, when everyone looks out for just themselves, we have peace, harmony and happiness all around? No, we have war, famine, abuse, hatred and despair. If you dissected every plague on modern society, outside of natural disasters and diseases (although this is a grey area, when you consider pharmaceutical companies, greed, deception, etc.—a subject for another book), you would find, at the core root of it, selfishness.

Why is there famine? Sure, areas experience drought, shortages, etc., but nine times out of ten, I would wager that there is one group of people or those in power hording all the resources for themselves. The same goes with power. How many wars have been started out of a lust for control and power? Also, how much ethnic and religious hatred have we seen in our past and still see today? What is at the root of hatred? Yep, you guessed it. Selfishness. You are so consumed by your own feelings of injury from another party or ingrained animosity that you don't consider, let alone act on a consideration, for them. I could go on and on, here.

Think about the opposite, now. If everyone truly desired the good of others, including themselves (but never at the expense of another's well-being), wouldn't the world be a better place? How about your country, state, community? What about your family, your personal relationships? Right now you're thinking, "Yeah, if only such and such a person would stop thinking about his/herself all the time, we'd be happy!"

Whoa, now! See what's happening there? Wouldn't it be best if we all focused on how we can change *our own* attitudes and *our own* actions?

I don't know about you, but I've experienced many an instance where I can almost step out of my body during a situation and look at my choices. I seem to intrinsically know that, if I react selfishly, things will end up badly, but if I act selflessly, it will turn out better. For example:

I come home from work, kids are climbing on me as if I'm walking playground equipment, I'm hungry, tired, a bit bedraggled after a stressful day, and my wife announces that it's cleaning night. Yes, indeed, family arrives from out of town tomorrow and we are at the necessity point of whipping the house into shape tonight. I have two choices at this point: 1) I can say, "Excuse me. I believe I've entered the wrong house. I don't know these children. I don't know any of you," and then run out as fast as I can, or 2) Whine and pout and do all in my power to avoid a little vacuuming and mopping. Okay, there's really a third choice, though I hate to admit. I can say, "Okay, I'm a bit tired and all that, but, let's hop to it!" Then, swallowing my grumpiness, putting on a little smile or whistle, I can get to work. If, in the past, I've chosen either option one or two, it's led to a night of tension, bitterness and mounting arguments. Option three, remarkably, ends up bringing more harmony into the household. So, I wonder, why is it always the hardest to choose option three?

Like I've said, we've got this natural disposition (or unnatural, you might say) to just look out for ourselves, to avoid suffering or hardship or inconvenience at all costs, even at the cost of hurting others.

I'm sure you can relate, if you take a close look at your life and situations similar to the one just described. When someone wants to come into your lane in traffic, why is there this urge to box them out or, worse yet, run them off the road and triumphantly close the four foot gap between you and the car ahead? When someone at the front of the line at the grocery store decides to search for a coupon, why do you suddenly, as if instinctively, let out a loud sigh and roll your eyes? When someone close to you asks you for a favor that requires a little sacrifice from you, why is your first reaction an inward groan and a quick evaluation of just how important that person is to you or how well your relationship would hold up if you flatly said "no?"

Maybe it's just me. Wow, I certainly hope not. That would be really embarrassing. I think we all share this selfish tendency, but, likewise, we also share this capacity for a true selflessness that is, in a word, love.

Food for Thought: *Do I live in a frantic, fruitless and frustrating pursuit of what will make me happy?*

Yes, I know that's a terribly overused word, but here I'm using it in a way that you don't hear on the soap operas or TV shows, or read about in the magazines. Here, I'm talking about the sincere desire for the utmost good of another person.

When we start to look at situations and other people in our lives as opportunities to show love, rather than to obtain a feeling of happiness from, the benefits are countless—and they flow both ways. Not only is it good for everyone around you, it's good for you, too. For one, it frees you from the desperate scramble for something you'll never get, i.e., true happiness from focusing on yourself, and it opens you up to a whole new world of peace and fulfillment.

Think about this for a moment. Some people lead their whole lives in perpetual pursuit of gratification, stuck in the same rut of extreme high, extreme low, "working for the weekend," for the next drinking spree, the next vacation getaway, only to find themselves more miserable when they return back to "normal life." It's like being on a fox hunt and never, ever, your entire life catching the fox. You see the bushy tail darting behind a tree, catch a fleeting glance of its clever eyes peering over a thicket, but you can never corner it or seize it. Maybe that's not the best example. Not many of us have been on those, and far too few have probably ever bellowed "Tally-ho!" for any reason or another. You should, though, really. It's quite fun. Take a moment to do that now. I'll wait. "Tally-ho!"

Okay, here's a better illustration: It's like misplacing a million dollar bill (we've all had one of those, right?). You search through your whole house, find some interesting things in the couch cushions, a farm of dust bunnies, Jimmy Hoffa, maybe, but not your money! You want the money! Every item of clothing, with every pocket, you have that small zing of exhilaration as you reach in, thinking *this* could be the time, this could be *it*. But you never find it. *Ever*.

How frustrating is that? Who wants to lead a life of constant frustration? Now, think of how liberating it would be if you just said, you know, I'm going to just forget the fox and enjoy the forest? Or, how much better would it be to say, hey, I'll Spring clean when the time comes, but I'm not going to waste years and years tearing apart my house, my entire life, looking for something that's just not going to be there? We can take a deep breath, relax our shoulders, maybe close our eyes, and then open them with the clear and freeing statement, "I will not be happy focusing on myself, so I'm going to stop doing that, right now."

My grandmother used to say, if you keep your expectations low, you'll always be happy with what you get. She, of course, was not referring to her cooking. There, you expected the best and you got it. If only life was as simple, pure and beautiful as a grandmother's kitchen. Maybe this is a good illustration because, if it was the classic, best-case example, that sacred ground was an aroma-filled place of self-giving love and true fulfillment. Love begets love, it's no secret. It just works.

Whoever said it's better to give than to receive knew exactly what he/she was talking about. I hope you've all experienced the rush of joy that comes over you when you give freely to another person without consideration for yourself. It's exhilarating. It's almost intoxicating. Now, imagine making this your primary focus and purpose in life. Go on. Stop and imagine it. You don't have to worry about chasing down self-gratifying experiences that always leave you empty. You accept that life is tough, but it's better when you focus on making others happy. Think about how freeing that would be. Yeah. That's what I'm talking about.

Okay, maybe you think I've gone nuts. Here are two more illustrations to help make this clear. First, from a story I was once told, "The Banquets of Long Utensils" (I'm guessing at the title, and I don't know the author). Yes, there were two grand banquets in two separate rooms, though both with the same amount of bounteous plates, platters and trays filled with the most delectable food you could imagine.

People sat on both sides of two endlessly long tables, ready to dig in. But, to their surprise, at both banquets, they found out that the utensils were at least four feet long! They were huge and very awkward. At one banquet, the people tried desperately to feed themselves with these utensils, but they could not. Food was falling everywhere, drinks spilling, glass breaking, the whole dinner getting ruined. Everyone grew irate and more and more savage as they fought to feed themselves with these long utensils. The result was chaos and despair.

Now, in the second banquet hall, a very simple solution was found. The people picked up their lengthy forks and spoons and began feeding the person across the table from them. It was remarkable. Everyone was happy and well-fed. It was paradise.

The second illustration is from my personal, all-time favorite movie, *It's a Wonderful Life*, directed by Frank Capra, starring Jimmy Stewart, Donna Reed, Lionel Barrymore and many other talented folks. The gist of the story: Here is this man, George Bailey, who from day one, lived to help others. It wasn't showy or overt. It was just who he was, and he didn't walk around all miserable about it. He had this sparkle in his eye. Sure, he never got anywhere, as far as money and success were concerned, and times got really rough at points, but what he had inside was the greatest treasure anyone could ask for: the joy that comes from loving and being loved in return. Okay, that was possibly one of the worst summaries of that timeless classic that you'll ever read. My advice: Watch it. If you don't have a tear at least lingering in your eye by the ending scene, then you must be a robot from the planet of Coldheartia.

Of course, this proposition of mine is a risky one. Give all your love away and trust that it will come back to you. Let's make that even worse: Be happy even if you don't ever "feel" that love come back to you from anyone or "fortune" or "fate," by way of accomplishments and accolades. Be happy, once you've served selflessly and they've laughed at you, spit at you, drug you into the street and beat you until you were blind. Why so extreme, you ask? Well, doesn't life feel that way sometimes? Isn't it at precisely this moment that you want to crawl out of the gutter and slip into a tub of hot fudge and ice cream? "Yes, food will comfort me when all else has let me down."

I'm speaking from experience here, and even at the writing of this book, I *still* do this at times! Yes, I'm not perfect. I don't always practice what I preach. I'm human. We all are (except for those of you who didn't cry at the end of my favorite movie mentioned above). Yet, it is precisely the fact that we're human that enables us to do what I've just outlined. Darwin's Survival of the Fittest is for the animals. Truly. Where, in that equation, does it mention submitting yourself to suffering for the good of another? No, you dominate if you want to last, if you want to survive, in his opinion. This is what the beasts of this planet do. But, we are not beasts. We are gifted with intellect and this amazing spark inside of us that *is* spirit and love.

You might say we were designed to be this way. Attribute it to a higher power, as most of the world's population does, or, if you want to say it was the way of evolution, you still cannot deny the fact that the world "works" when we love others, not when we dominate out of love for self.

Here, my friends, is the rub. No, a masseuse is not showing up at your door, now! Focus, people! I've arrived at the crux* of my argument: If we are meant to be selfless givers, we will not find true happiness until we live this way. Is a horse happy if it is never allowed to run? Can an artist live if you spill out all of his paint and break his brushes? If you take a dolphin and put it in a barn with chickens . . . I think you get my point!

Okay, we've discovered that our looks are transitory, our health fragile, and happiness, the emotion, is fleeting. So, we can't find true happiness in these. Maybe, at this point, if we're not distracted by the latest commercial on TV, we're willing to admit that this whole "selflessness = joy" theory has some merit and may be worth a try. So, the question remains, how on this everloving Earth do we break our ingrained, unhealthy attitude toward food and find the strength to live life as we were meant to live it?

Read on, my friends. Read on.

---

* Don't you just love the word "crux?" It's such a cool word. Crux. Look at it, so economical in letters, yet verbose and poignant at the same time. I think I'll start a rock band, despite my utter lack of musical talent, just so I can name it Crux. But, I digress . . .

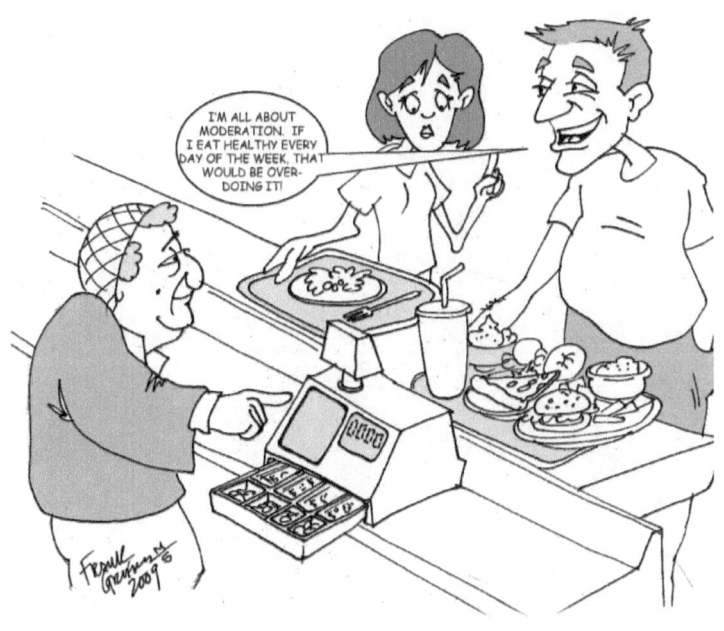

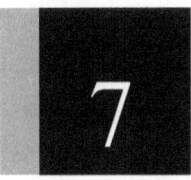

How do I do this!?
(Time to roll up our sleeves)

Step One: <u>Recognize the problem</u>.
Great! You've already done that! One step down, baby!
Only a few more to go.

      Just to make sure though, repeat after me (and with
me): "I use food to make me happy, and that's my
problem." Now, let's repeat that phrase and include any
other thing that we try to fill the void with, i.e., our
appearance, health, loved ones, drugs, sex, alcohol, power,
etc. Take time with this, focus on the problem. Here's my
list: food, writing (ha,ha!), coffee, and time. Time, you ask?
What do I mean by that? Let me clarify by saying: *my* time.
I'm talking about this pervading thought that, if I could
only have some time to myself to do what I want to do,
whatever it is, I'll be happy. Of course, if I keep on this
track, ironically, someday I'll have all the time I want . . .
because I'll be alone, and I'll be miserable.

What's your list?

Step Two:

Recognize the solution. I know you may not entirely agree or are convinced yet about this one, but, please try it with me, give it a shot. If you do agree, great! Shout it out from the rooftops! Join me in saying, "Selfishness brings despair. Giving of myself brings true happiness!"

Step Three: Take a break and eat a fudge brownie. Just kidding, there. This next step is crucial, and it's common to most rehabilitation programs: **Admit that you cannot do this alone.**

Form a support group. If it's your spouse, great-- a close friend, a men's group, women's group, your dog— perfect. Really, most animals don't overeat, do they? They eat enough to satisfy and survive. Unless, of course, they've been around us so much that they've picked up our unhealthy habits. Bottom line, find someone or a group to talk this all through with and, most importantly, hold each other accountable in making the positive changes needed. Okay, so maybe your pet won't work here. Not unless your cat can jump up on the table, pin down your ice cream spoon and say, "Hey, what did we talk about, huh? What're you doin' here?!"

We're not supposed to go through this alone. We are meant to help each other out, to share our trials and to support each other. Reach out to someone (distribute copies of this book, if need be. *Shameless, I know*), and you'll find that people are hungry for this type of bonding and aide in life.

Now, I actually skipped the first part of step three. It's fundamental, from my experience and that of countless others, in order to heal and find strength to live the way we are meant to live: Recognize that you need help from on high. Am I talking about the guru on top of the mountain? No, I'm talking about God, or Allah, or The Higher Power, whatever name you attribute to the guiding power and source of goodness in the universe.

NOTE: The following is what I sincerely believe. I told you I wouldn't be pushy about my specific beliefs, and I'll try not to, but I can't sincerely suggest the way to a healthy relationship with food, let alone true happiness, and leave this out. I really don't recommend this, but you can, by all means dismiss the following and move on to the next step, trying to go this alone. Here's the deal. At least read it, consider it, and keep an open mind. You've stuck with me this far. What have you got to lose?

I'm trying to be sensitive to all beliefs, here, but, in order to move on, I have to be more particular, and so I'll touch on this from my own personal experience. I have learned, in my lifetime, that I can't do this alone. I need God. Yes, I've said it. You thought the ad execs were angry before? Oh, yeah. The "Get Michael" encampment just got a lot more crowded now.

Why is it that people get so touchy when you bring up God? Is it because they're afraid you're going to try to convert them or force your "rules" on them? Whatever happened to free and open discussion, to learning from one another? I feel that the harsh reaction comes more from an ingrained mentality that's become the very fabric of modern man's identity, especially the American person. Quite simply, it's this: I am a self made man. I can do anything, build anything, make it anywhere on my own. Isn't this what our great nation was founded on, after all, rugged individualism? Um, no. Look at any of the original writings of our Founding Fathers that haven't been "censored" by school boards, and you'll see these noble statesmen down on their knees, literally, pleading with their God for help to make sure they started this country off right. If you look closely at all of our nation's major monuments in D.C., you'll see inscriptions, prayers chiseled out for all time, asking God for protection, strength and guidance.

Food for Thought: *Do you ever feel like you're seen more as a demographic member than a person?*

You ask why I keep bringing up the ad executive? One word: consumerism. It feeds off the "I need" and, mostly, the "I want, I want, I want!" mentalities. If people start thinking less about themselves, they'll start spending less frivolously. Oh, no! The economy would collapse! Forget about it, if people get religion! That's the ultimate danger. Those darn fanatics do crazy things like sell their property and give to the poor; they fast, and, oh brother, they abstain from sex at times! Well, there goes the entire advertising paradigm!

Okay, trying not to get too far off topic, here. Let's bring this back in. And please realize that one of the most successful alcoholism rehab programs in the world, Alcoholics Anonymous, includes this important factor. Remember how we talked about food being the next legal drug? It has been proven that people caught in the throngs of addiction find more hope and success when they come to realize that they have help from above-- that it's not all up to them. If it was all up to me, I'd give up now, because I know just how incompetent I am at times, and I can't possibly see or comprehend the big picture, thus rightly putting things in their proper place. Heck, I can't even decide what to eat for lunch sometimes without taking fifteen minutes!

I'll be the first to admit that, some days, I can't stand myself. Maybe it's how I look or feel, or I've acted like a jerk, but, I have to say, I find immeasurable comfort in knowing that God loves me more than I could possibly imagine. I'm not going to try and prove His existence here (read C.S. Lewis' *Mere Christianity* for this, among other great books); I'm just going to say that having a relationship with Him has helped me to put my life into focus, and it gives me the strength to get through the most difficult of times. Honestly, I don't know how people get by without it.

In my faith, I am able to overcome so many hurdles that, otherwise, are very difficult, if not impossible for me to do. Believe me, I've tried it alone! Take forgiveness. How can we function, let alone love selflessly when there's hatred in our hearts? It just doesn't work. We've all been there. Maybe some are still there. Knowing that God forgives me, and gives me the grace to forgive because it is the right thing to do for me, for the other person, for our world, I can do it! Sure, not perfectly, and it takes time, sometimes, but, again, I know I have support in this, supernatural support.

Remember how we talked about the improbability of finding happiness all the time from another person? God, being God, will never let me down and will always be there for me. This is good news. This is great news! The same goes with support. That person or group we might cling to during this process is going to disappoint at times. That's just the way it is. It's a great solace to me knowing that, at the end of the day, heck, at any moment in the day, I've got a source of truth and sustenance right there with me to help me stay positive and on track.

This leads me to an action item within this important step: PRAY." "Here he goes," you say, "lassoing out with the Rosary beads, trying to reel me in!"

I'm not pushing, I'm hoping to share here, that's all. Here's what I'm saying: Just like we have to constantly remind ourselves that we are valuable for who we are, not what we look like or do, etc., we can't just acknowledge a loving God exists and then move on.

What is prayer? Simply put, it's talking with God; it's building a relationship. Well, you say, isn't it a little one-sided, since he generally doesn't talk back? Ask anyone in a close relationship with their Maker and you'll hear that He does talk back, through sacred writings, love letters as it were, to lead us to him and help us find fulfillment, through the beauty and wonder of nature, through the quiet whisperings in our souls, and through the people in our lives, to name more than a few ways.

So, cast out your net. Throw out a prayer. You'll be surprised at what you reel back in. For me, like I said, it's been the very foundation and nourishment with which I try to live a selfless, joyful and purposeful life.

What exactly is the purpose behind my life? It's that "L" word again. I bet you can guess it.

And, remember, since we're not meant to base our lives on a search for the feeling of happiness, here's a key directive: Don't expect or come to depend on spiritual highs or ecstasies, as they are called. Many people start a spiritual journey and are filled

> **Food for Thought:**
> *Why am I here? Is it to give or to take?*

with such wonderful feelings that, when these drop away, they believe it couldn't have been real or that God has abandoned them. It only makes sense to me that, if God wants us in the trenches loving despite our pain, through our trials, He's going to train and condition us to do so.

Some people, like Mother Theresa, I've read, went through years, if not decades of spiritual dryness, where they felt nothing, yet they still persevered. What carried them through? For some, it was the memory of one moment of spiritual ecstasy that sustained them in the valley of darkness, while for others, it was simply knowing what was true and right and sticking to it until the end. If we can't hope that they saw the fruits of this in the last, what can we pin our hopes to in this world?

Now, I've already justified the necessity of loving self-sacrifice for a better life and world, but what about this thing called suffering? What about the earthquakes, murders, hurricanes, typhoons, kidnappings and the host of innumerable afflictions this world has to offer? We can't discuss adjusting our attitude toward food as it relates to true happiness without facing these issues, can we?

So many people can't reconcile that a loving God would allow seemingly needless pain and suffering. Therefore, since all of the bad stuff exists, then God simply cannot, or at least a loving one anyway. And who wants to even consider an unloving god? I'll spend just a few more moments on this, because, really, it is an anchor point for me and so many others. If you don't come to terms with this, so often everything else falls apart and you're cut loose and drifting in cold, frightening uncertainty.

Here's what I believe. You can take it or leave it. Of course, if this answer doesn't satisfy you, and sure, it may not without further consideration, reading, contemplation and, yes, prayer (why *not* ask the One with all the answers?), then please keep digging and searching for a better understanding of this Truth that will give you peace. You will find it. For now, consider this: God loves us. We're starting to understand that love *is* the way. So, it makes sense that, if God truly wants our perfect good, He would want for us to love each other and Him completely, right? The question is, he's God, right, so why doesn't he just make people love? That would take care of all of the selfishness that leads to so much sorrow and suffering, right? Well, maybe. But, then it wouldn't be love.

"But, you just said--! And I just said--!" "Yes, but did you just say you said what you said you said when I said what I said you said I said?" (Sorry, had to have some fun, there.)

Okay, it comes down this: Authentic love is one that is freely given. Forcing someone to love makes it a response to oppression. Designing someone so they have no choice but to love makes it a programmed response, hardly a free gift. As we've seen on both a personal and global scale, the decision to love or not to love is inherent in every choice we make, every positive or negative outcome, and so, taking away that choice, or free will, as some call it, what you have left is really a world full of robots. We wouldn't even know we were showing love to

[93]

others. We wouldn't be thinking rationally, that's for sure, because every decision would be made for us.

Now, I'm not saying that bad choices and suffering exist so that we could know the difference between love and hate. The freedom to choose between the two is the greatest gift and privilege. Unfortunately, so many times we fail in both major and minor ways with this choice. Hence, the hurting of others and ourselves. But, can you see now that it really cannot be any other way and still hold the possibility for life-giving and transforming love? With this great gift of freedom, comes that word we often wish we could ignore: responsibility.

Now, I could move on, here, but I feel that would be a disservice, not to mention sneaky on my part. I talked about suffering that resulted from bad choices resulting from the ability to choose, without which we would have no love and true happiness, but I didn't mention the suffering that results from storms, quakes, disease, and other things that are not caused by a person's decision.

"So there you have it, Mr. Smartypants," you say. "Give me a good explanation for how a loving God could let countless innocents suffer from these things!"

Well, you're probably not going to like the answer, but here it is: faith. It all ties back to my faith that God is preparing for me and everyone else something so much greater in that afterlife place we like to call Heaven, Paradise, or, simply being in the arms of the One we love, forever. This world is a dangerous place, no doubt about it,

[94]

but if we choose to love and be close to Him in this life, then, in whatever way we leave this world, at whatever time, we'll be with Him in the next. And, there will be no more tears, no more suffering.

"Fine," you say. "But, do we just view hardship and pain in life as necessary evils and only that?"

No, I believe the role of suffering in our daily lives is integral to everything we've talked about and everything we're trying to accomplish. And, if a picture could paint a thousand words, let's go back to the Sistine Chapel and look up at the depiction of Christ, the son of God, dying on the cross. For so many, this is a contradiction that can't be reconciled. For me, it makes perfect sense. It is the ultimate gift of love, God atoning for our sins for all time, and, at the same time, showing us the way to happiness, showing us the redemptive power in suffering. If we don't rebel against it with bitterness, the pain in our lives can be looked at as an opportunity to become better lovers. It trains us to sacrifice and to accept hardship for the good of others.

We already know that focusing just on ourselves leads to destruction on a personal and global scale. It only follows, then, that dying to self, would lead to life. Christ's suffering models this perfectly, and our own suffering can help us to defeat selfishness in our lives on a daily basis. The better we become at this, the happier we are and the better off our families are and our world becomes.

I know this is pretty deep stuff and requires a lot more thought and reflection, but I hope you can see now at least how my relationship with God gives me purpose, understanding, perspective and strength for the task of loving. I could go into how I've been touched personally in so many ways, blessed in more ways than I can count (and deserve), and how I find daily help and nourishment in the particular gifts my faith has to offer, but that would take too long and, hey, this isn't about me, is it!? Let's put the focus back on you.

Really, to satisfy step three, I believe finding someone or a group to support you is key, and, as far as a relationship with the Absolute, if you're not already deep into one, a great start is recognizing you need Heavenly Help, praying for it throughout your day, and beginning the search process to get to know God better. Really, what relationship lasts, if there isn't good communication, along with healthy discovery? And guess what? He's always happy to hear from you, no matter what.

Okay, whew! Moving on with the practical action items in living a life of true happiness!

Step Four: Eat right.

Step Five: Take a blue beetle by the wings—Wait, what's that you say? You're not happy with how I treated step four? Well, come on, now! Did I ever claim I was the diet guru? By diet, I mean, the food you eat every day. I guess I should go into it further, let you know my philosophy, though it's not all that original, I'm warning you.

Here it is: Moderation. You knew I was going to say that, didn't you? Something told you I wasn't going to go to some low carb or high carb, or low protein, or high fiber plan, didn't it? Maybe it's my upbringing. Maybe it's my experience. I find, though, that if I stick to that fun food triangle, include protein, veggies, dairy, carbs and fruit in my meals, and I'm not overdoing it in any category, then I'm on the right track.

I suggest taking a course on nutrition at a local community college. There's so much to learn. Now, I said I wouldn't adhere to any of the trendy plans out there, but, without naming names, I think the calorie counting ones are pretty good because they boil down to being aware of what you're putting into your body. Of course, every time I see those commercials that say you can eat whatever you want as long as you don't exceed your daily point allowance, I think of myself using up all my points at breakfast by eating a chocolate cake. Then what would I do?

I'm learning, as I get older, that moderation is the key in so many areas. If I work too much, it's bad. If I exercise too much, something starts to break down. If I eat too much, I start putting on unnecessary pounds. So, the answer's simple, right? Don't eat too much!

And, for heaven's sake, don't you dare touch that dessert! Sweets are the enemy!

No, see, I don't adhere to that. Moderation applies to treats, too. I think where so many diets go wrong is that they make the person feel like they are depriving themselves of what they truly want the most, and then, when they fall off the wagon, it's usually into a binge pool.

The way I look at it and try to live is that I can have a sweet thing, now and then, once or twice a week, or more, depending on the occasion or how disciplined I feel I need to be at the time. And, "a little dab will do ya." Just one slice of cake should suffice, instead of two or three. One scoop of ice cream is a nice treat on a Friday night; a twelve gallon sundae tub is really not necessary. I mean, do we really need to pour it on like that? The law of diminishing returns almost always comes into play, like we discussed in Chapter 3. After a while, you're plowing through the rest of your dessert without much pleasure, just to conquer it, and, when it's been defeated, you're almost always sick in the end. A little bit of something sweet to satisfy the craving works for me.

And, you know what, fruit is really the best, I've found. Grapes! They're awesome, oblong, bursting bubbles of refreshing enjoyment. You can't beat that! And pineapple, watermelon—these are amazingly sweet and all natural. I've always said, God makes the best desserts. Try including fruit at the end of each meal and see that your craving for something sweet is practically gone. Soon, you'll find that sugary, fattening sweets aren't all that important to you anymore (stop laughing, it's true).

So, eat right, using moderation. Easier said than done, right? That's where we come to the real Step Five: Take it moment by moment.

It's pretty common, at least with me, that, just because I know something, doesn't mean I do it every time. To say right now, "Food does not make me happy," and put down the book and never remind yourself of that fact would be foolish. Remember, we're not robots. We have choices, darn it all, so here's the way to confront each food choice throughout the day:

When you're deciding what to cook for a meal, or buy at the grocery store, or whether to go for the fast-food, remind yourself, "Food does not make me happy."

When you settle down after a hard day, and you start thinking about feeding your craving with too much of something sweet or unnecessary, repeat, in your head, "Food does not make me happy."

When they wheel the dessert cart past you at the restaurant and you find yourself clutching onto the handle and unable to let go, repeat after me, calmly and slowly, "Food does not make me happy." Then, let go and return to your table.

I promise you, that feeling like you can't live without the fudge swirl pound cake *will pass!* The feeling that you just won't be happy unless you're sucking on your nightly milkshake *will go away*. Force yourself through the tough craving moment or moments, and then congratulate yourself for having won the battle. And, oh yeah, be sure and keep yourself from strangling the people around you who are partaking in the treat you passed up!

[99]

It always seems to work this way: The times when you're attempting to cut back on sweets, your spouse or someone close to you shows up eating a half gallon of ice cream.

"Mmmm! This is soooo good! This might just be the best ice cream I've ever tasted in my life!"

"Hey, uh, could you not eat that right in my face?" you say, trying to keep the tone of your voice civil.

"What are you talking about? I'm not right in your face!"

"You're sitting on my lap waving each spoonful under my nose!"

"Oh, sorry."

The great thing is, you'll start to find that, the more little victories you have, the easier the next battle becomes. It's like weight-lifting. You're training yourself to avoid what's bad for you and to accept all the good. Soon, you'll be like Mr. or Mrs. Universe and, everywhere you go, people will hurl donuts and pastries at you, but they'll just bounce off of you and you won't even know they're there.

Those are the essential steps. Not too complicated, huh?

- We know food can't make us happy.
- We know only love can, but we can't do it alone.
- We know we need to eat right and confront the temptation to not eat right on an instance by instance basis.

We also know that this is one area that oversimplifying just won't do. As promised, what follows is a chapter chock full of helpful tips and strategies to fighting the <u>good food fight</u>, day by day.

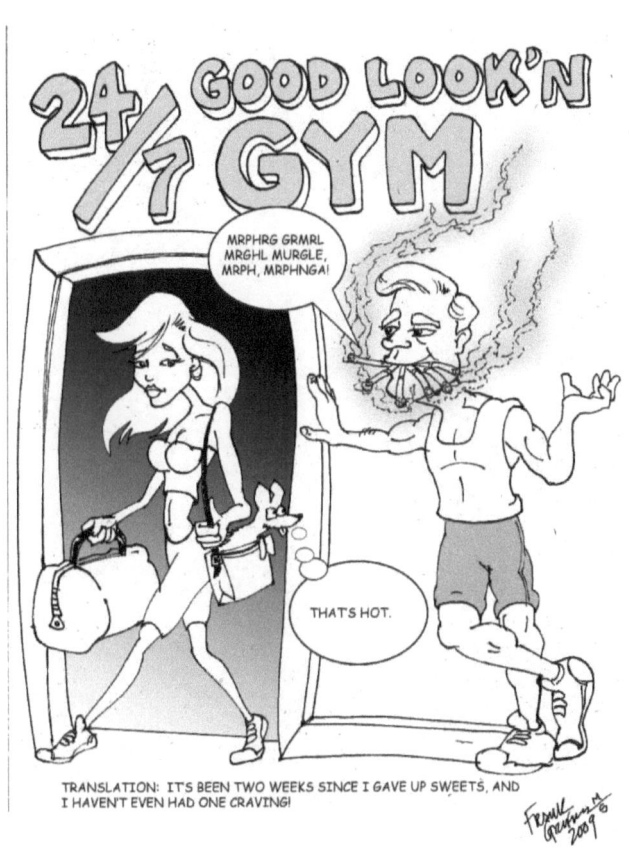

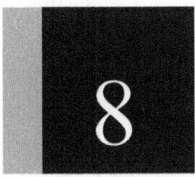

8

Holidays are Not Evil
(and other useful things to remember)

Why do we gain weight around the holidays? Is it because we want to be ripe, jolly old elves like Santa? Is it because, due to poor weather conditions in most places, there's less to do outdoors and more to do indoors, like bake and eat?

FOOD TIP #1:

Treat the holidays like any other time of year, food-wise. Bake all you want for the little ones and for company, but moderation, moderation, moderation when it comes to how many you snatch when the lights are low.

"Daddy, Santa ate all twenty cookies that you left for him!"

"Yes, and I almost made myself sick! I mean, er, I'm sure he loved them!"

You can't avoid the extra treats around the holidays, the smell of ginger and cinnamon in the air, or the candies and cakes that arrive at your door. Just, don't eat them all! Distribute them to family, friends and neighbors. Remind yourself, I don't need food to make my holidays happy! I have the true meaning of the season to sustain me, and a bottle of Jack Daniels! No, no. (See tip #3 about this!).

Whatever you do, don't try to cut out all treats and sweets from your holiday experience. Enjoy this time of year! Food can be play a part in all of it. Just not the lead role. Have that cup of cocoa with your kids or other loved ones. Just don't pile in two hundred of those seductively fluffy and delightfully buoyant sugar puffs we like to call marshmallows. And, you know, I wish people would stop calling them marsh-"mellows." Maybe I wouldn't have misspelled that word in my 3rd grade spelling bee and could've gone on to be a champion, a contender! (Sorry, I'll save comments like that for my counselor next time).

Final note on this: the holidays tend to be busy, stressful times (unfortunately), so it's key to still do your best to stick as closely as possible to your regular exercise routine. And, since we often have family and friends in around us, why not involve them? Go on a walk together or throw together some teams and play your favorite sport.

"Dad, we're gonna toss the old pigskin around. Come on!"

"I can't! I'm stuffed. I'm like a piñata! The kids got out the wiffle ball bat from the garage and I hid in the pantry for like an hour."

"That's the whole point! We're all full. We need to work it off. Besides, Uncle Al's playing, and we all know you're just looking for a chance to drag his face through the mud."

"Okay, now you're talkin'!"

FOOD TIP #2:

<u>Get a hobby</u>. Really, distraction is sometimes one of the best weapons. If you feel yourself getting into a serious craving, after you've told yourself, "Food does not make me happy," you can turn to your whittling knife and continue your personal rendition of Mount Rushmore in your living room.

Note here, that sleeping is *not* a hobby! I've gone through this before. Sometimes the temptation to splurge is so bad and the withdrawal so strong that I just want the night to be over.

"Goodnight, honey! I'm turning in!"

"Michael, it's six o'clock! The kids are still awake."

"Great! They can tuck *me* in for a change! And, can you tell them to bring me a glass of water?"

Learn another language, grow a garden, take a cooking class (really!), or pull out those pens and paints you've had packed away for so long. Doing something constructive like this with your time will not only keep your mind off food, it will be satisfying and productive, too!

In fact, if you look back at all the great inventions of the past, you'll see that they usually occurred when the inventor was on a diet. Why do you think Ben Franklin was outside, in the middle of a thunderstorm, flying a kite? He wasn't allowed to go bowling with the rest of the Founding Fathers? He had a death wish? No, it was to avoid watching his wife enjoy another helping of pudding and crumpets, that's why!

Eli Whitney invented the cotton harvester he named the cotton gin. Cotton. Gin. Hmm. What was he trying to avoid, do you think?

Marconi and the radio? Look at the guy's name, for crying out loud! Tell me you're not thinking of pasta! I'm sure he was trying not to!

FOOD TIP #3:

Don't replace one addiction with another.

"Bob, have you lost weight? You look like you're trimming up!"

"Mmmphhhhergurglehmph."

"Bob, I can't hear you. You have five lit cigarettes in your mouth!"

Seriously, the temptation is unmistakable. When you've been filling the void with one thing, and you take that away, your instinct is to fill it with something else. Cigarettes and coffee are prime examples, because, yeah, they're legal and they're not very fattening, like beer or peppermint schnapps. If we find ourselves leaning in this direction, or buying a portable espresso machine that we can strap to our backs, we need to reevaluate.

You might say, "Now, come on! Don't take away everything I love at once! I can't stand it! I'll go insane. I'll give up! I'll go back to my old ways, I tell you! You don't know me!"

My answer is, if you're anything like me, then I know you. I never said this would be easy. But, again, shifting your attitude toward a healthier and happier tomorrow will help in all this. If food won't make us happy, it only follows that no other substance or obsession on this earth will.

Your response might be, "Hey I don't smoke or drink to be happy. I just want to take the edge off, relax a little." For this, I tip my hat to the advertising companies behind the cigarette and alcohol ads. You know, they really know their stuff.

You don't see beer billboards depicting guys with pregnant guts, glued to a couch and a TV with their wives handing them divorce papers. No, you see fit and attractive men and women smiling, laughing and having a good time! Same with cigarette ads. They don't portray people with yellow or blackened teeth. They don't show people on respirators or dying of cancer. No, they show cool, hip, relaxed, in style.

We can't substitute one bad thing or habit for another. If we're really going to do this, then we have to do it all the way. It's like saying, "I'm really going to start exercising from now on, because it's good for me, reduces stress, helps keep me in shape— but, just my left leg.

That's enough. The rest of me? That would be too extreme!"

No, we've got to go all the way with this.

FOOD TIP #4:
Make an effort on a daily, hour by hour basis, to not focus on yourself.

Here's another catchphrase I've found to be helpful. "It's not about me. It's not about me." Sometimes, I go around thinking that I'm all that matters; that I'm the star of this epic movie called "Present Time in the World as We Know It." The truth is, it's an ensemble cast. It's about the people right there in my house, in my community, and all across the globe, all of us working together.

What usually helps with this is visiting a poor country, poor part of town or stopping to hear about someone going through a very tough situation in life. Maybe they are terribly sick. Maybe they're losing a loved one. Listening, reflecting on the lives of these people usually makes me want to kick myself afterwards for ever complaining about my "problems."

In other words, we all have to fight the "poor me" syndrome. It's everywhere. It's deep inside me. It's in my relationships. Do you find yourself doing this with your spouse or loved one, comparing your days to see who's had the worst one?

"You won't believe how crazy my day was!"

"Your day!? You don't even want to know about mine!"

"We had a toner spill in the office."

"I had throw-up all over the kitchen."

"I got a flat tire."

"I got pulled over by a cop!"

"My head hurts!"

"Yeah? Well, my head was abducted by the kids hours ago, and they're holding it hostage!"

We waste so much time trying to outdo the other when it would probably be best if we each said, "Sorry you had such a rough day. What can I do for you?"

"Yes," you say, "and a flock of pigs would, at that moment, fly right over our house. My husband would never say this," you might add, or, "My wife would sooner die than acknowledge me!"

All I can say is, start with you. You do it and keep on doing it. Whether you see some immediate returns or not, I promise, it will pay off in ways you never dreamed possible.

I have seen it work. If I can remind myself to stop judging my happiness on what I can get and start investing it more in what I can give, I find that my family's happier, my work prospers, and I'm not futilely trying to fill the void all the time. I'm satisfied with living as I was meant to live. When I do this, it's really the best of times. Of course, I can only count on one hand how often I've truly lived in this state of mind . . . But, I promise to keep trying. How about you?

FOOD TIP #5:

<u>Take the money you would normally spend on excess food or treats and give it to someone in need</u>. Sponsor a poverty-stricken child across the globe, or help a local family down on their luck. I'm no sociologist or scientist, but, all I'm saying is, you want to solve world hunger, this might be a good place to start.

Again, this is something that usually fits the easier-said-than-done category. I'm ashamed to admit this, but I'm one of those people who become so wrapped up in the everyday needs/wants of life, that I tend to forget about doing the things I feel most passionate about. Why is it I can squeeze in the time to pick up a treat, but not help someone out?

"Honey, there was all this traffic on the way home from the store because of this big accident. It was awful!"

"Really? Was anyone hurt?"

"I don't know, but our ice cream's almost completely melted now! Can you believe our luck?"

Shameful, huh?

A good idea would be to put a jar out in the home where the money I would use to get something sweet could go into, and then, at a particular point each month, I could empty the jar and rush off to a bakery—no, make a donation to aid those in need.

FOOD TIP #6:

<u>After you tell yourself that "Food does not make me happy," be sure to open your eyes to the pure and simple things in this life that *do* bring you joy</u>.

Maybe it's a smile exchanged with a stranger, or your child's tiny hand in yours, or watching a hummingbird dance around a flower. Sure, these may be passing moments, but they are glimpses of the eternal joy that awaits us and, I believe, rays of encouragement in this oftentimes bleak and cruel world. If we let them, they can lift us up each day-- but we've got to let them!

Cherish the people in your life. Listen to them like you never have before. Enjoy each other's company. Let go of bitterness, and learn to minimize petty fights or squabbles. Really, our time here is so fleeting. Do we really want to spend it greedily shoving our faces and constantly bickering with those close to us? What kind of legacy are we building?

How about a legacy of love?

Anyone? Any takers?

FOOD TIP #7:

<u>Don't stock up on sweets</u>! Nothing stops you from overindulging in sweets more than not having them in your freezer, fridge or cupboards! Sure, it's tough with parents, when you want to have stuff available for the kiddies.

Two things on this: One, there are plenty of healthy snacks and treats to give your children. Wouldn't it be great to start them off with good habits early on in life when it comes to what they eat? Two, kids are kids and they shouldn't have to suffer because you're trying to resist urges. So, if you need to have some candy around or sweets, don't pick *your* favorites! Pick something you don't particularly care for, and keep that around.

"Kids, gather around for a treat!"

"Yeah!"

"Chocolate-covered grasshoppers coming right up!"

"Noooo!"

Obviously, this is extreme, and may not always work. You may want to start off with chocolate-covered ants first.

Oh yeah, and give your keys to a designated security person who won't let you drive out to the store in the middle of the night to take solace in your favorite frozen food section.

FOOD TIP #8:

The reward mentality needs to go. Have you ever found yourself thinking or saying, "I deserve a treat!" after a long day? What are we, dogs?! I mean, really! If we got through the day without killing anyone or losing our job, does that mean we're entitled to a food reward? Yes, I'm sure you can roll over, too, and beg and shake hands. That's not gonna cut it, though. Please, get up off the floor. You're embarrassing yourself.

Shouldn't the reward be simply in the intrinsic value of a job having been done well?

A good thing to do when you find yourself in this frame of mind is to think of a starving child in Africa. What does he or she *deserve*? Seriously, we need to take that five dollars a week that we spend on a pint of ice cream and sponsor that child (remember tip #5?). It's money much better spent. And then we could reward ourselves with satisfaction that does not fade along with the sugar high, but with lasting fulfillment by living how we were meant to live.

Okay, I see you begging with your paws in the air and tongue out. You're not getting the treat right now, so you might as well give up!

FOOD TIP #9:

Hunger pains are good. I don't know about you, but at times I've fallen into the trap of thinking, whenever I get the slightest pang of hunger in my stomach, I need to put food in my mouth. But really, we don't need to be eating all day long. We can stand to feel a little hunger between meals.

Small, healthy snacks in between meals are good, but these shouldn't be every ten minutes!

People of faiths all around the world do what's called fasting, going for a period of time without eating.

[115]

Some rites of passage into adulthood would include going for days without eating. I can't go two hours. Does that mean I'm still a child?

Spiritually speaking, people use it as a form of prayer and sacrifice, and also as a way to show that they are not dependent on food, but on a higher power. Gandhi used fasting as a way of peaceful protest to bring about political change in India, once again showing that there is a higher ideal at stake that is worth sacrificing for. I'm not suggesting you lock yourself in your office and hold off from eating until you can convince your boss to give you that promotion you've been working for. But, consider at least, that it's okay to be hungry at times, maybe even beneficial.

That being said . . .

FOOD TIP #10:

<u>Don't starve yourself</u>! I can never understand when people say, "I went all day without eating!" This is just startling to me. I mean, if I don't eat for a long time, my body tells me, point blank, "Hi, Michael. Yeah, you feel that headache? How about that bit of wobbliness in the knees, not to mention your mounting grumpiness? Eat!"

Some people think they're going to make progress in losing weight if they skip a meal or two a day. Wrong-o! It's been proven that your body, if not fed appropriately at least three times a day, will take whatever food comes in and convert it into fat, thinking that it's in a crisis situation and that it needs to store up for it. Funny, isn't it, when your own body has the last laugh at your expense?

FOOD TIP #11:

Drink lots of water. Did you know that our cells are made up of something like 95% water? How amazing is that? How we don't just melt away with the rain or disappear when we dive into a swimming pool, I'll never know! The point here is that so many people don't realize just how much we need water and lots of it throughout our day.

A lot of negative ways we feel at times, i.e., fatigue, headaches, agitation, can be solved by a nice, tall glass of water. Will wine do, you ask? No. Your favorite cola? Sorry.

"But, it's got water in it!" you shout back, like a pouting child.

"Yes, and lots of other stuff that's not good for you, and defeats the purpose."

Here's a good one: "I don't like the taste of water!"

"What taste?! It's water! It doesn't have any taste!"

I just spent some time in China, recently, and it struck me at dinnertime, while watching a fellow American struggle with the fact that there was no soy sauce available for the plain, white rice in front of us, WE AMERICANS CAN'T HAVE ANYTHING PLAIN!

I don't know where this came from, but we desperately have to put stuff on top of stuff! A burger isn't good unless it has mustard, ketchup, special sauce, not-so-special sauce, 1000 Island dressing, ad infinitum on it. Plain vanilla ice cream? No way! That's like an insult to most red-blooded Americans. We need hot fudge, caramel, nuts, whipped cream, and anything else sweet and oozing on top.

We may eat a big salad for a meal and be proud of ourselves, ignoring the fact that we drowned it out with fattening Ranch dressing, bacon bits and chunks of heath bars in it. Okay, it's not that bad, but why is it that we are so "taste-dependant?"

Try a bowl of plain white rice with your meal sometime. It's actually quite good. Simple, pure and good.

For the people who say, "I just can't drink water because I don't like how it tastes," I have one reply: "Do you like the way air tastes?"

"Well, I, er, um—"

We need air to live. It's the same with water: good, clean and simple H_2O. It replenishes us, keeps us hydrated, gives us energy, and, if you're fighting some hunger pains, it's a great way to help hold you over until it's time to eat. In fact, I'm doing that right now. It was an hour until lunch when I started writing this segment. I felt the old gnawing in the gut and thought, "Maybe just a cracker or two, or a cereal bar," but, instead, and I'll admit, somewhat begrudgingly, I opened a bottle of water and started drinking. Five minutes to go until lunch and I think I'm gonna make it! If not—if they find me sprawled out, too weak to open the plastic wrap around a cracker-- tell my wife and kids . . . I love them . . .

FOOD TIP #12:

<u>Don't stay up late</u>! You may ask what this has to do with losing weight, and my answer is two-fold: One, what happens when you normally stay up late? Yes, you guessed it. You start to get hungry again. Maybe you're trying to watch a movie or stay awake for the late show when you're totally exhausted, and what do you do? You make yourself a sandwich or grab for the bag of chips, or, like me, you might go for the bowl of cereal you have no business having six or seven hours before it was meant to be had. When you stay up late, you usually munch, eating more calories than your body really needed for the day.

Secondly, it has been documented that people who do not get enough sleep have a very hard time losing weight and, oftentimes gain weight more easily. Not sure, physically how this works, but I know from reading it, and from experience, that it's true.

For me, I need to examine why I'm staying up late. Is it because I don't want the next day to come? Why? Is it fear? Is it depression? Will staying up late and making myself tired the next day really help with either of these?

Is it because things have finally quieted down and I want some leisure time with my wife or time for myself? This is fine, but it needs to be in moderation, just like anything else. We go through these "defy the week" periods, renting a movie on Sunday night and staying up late, scoffing at the upcoming school/work day. Is this really the best way to start off the week, tired and grumpy? Or, would it be better to do something brief, but fun, call it a night, and then wake up fresh and ready to face the next day's challenges with rest on our side?

Here is a list of brief, but fun things you can do with your spouse (besides the obvious one! Ha, ha. I know what you're thinkin'!):

- ❖ Card game. This is always fun. Unless, of course, one of you is extremely competitive and can't stand losing.
- ❖ Catalogue your CD collection. Okay, maybe not.
- ❖ Watch one episode of a funny show both of you enjoy. One episode-- not two, three or four!
- ❖ Talk. (I can't believe I just suggested this.) However, if you talk, not into the wee small hours of the morning, but for a good half hour or so, discussing the upcoming week's events or trials, this is a great way to unite together. And, closing with a prayer together is an amazing way to bring healing and grace into your marriage.
- ❖ Read together. Whatever happened to this? Are we so technologically dependant that we can't sit in bed like people used to do, and read? Then, you can lean over and share what you've gleaned. You can have a mutual, gleaning experience. Doesn't that sound fun?
- ❖ Laundry! Nothing spells fun better than folding clothes together! However, something like this can be a

bonding experience, where you work together to meet a need, so one person doesn't feel like the burden is always on them alone.

❖ Joke around and laugh together. This is simply the best. Sometimes, you know each other so well you can get on a laugh track that sends you giggling into the night. These are some great memories that are healthy, positive and priceless. Share an embarrassing moment from the day, or a joke you heard. Be open. Be silly, disarming, playful. If you can't do this with each other, who can you do it with? If you haven't before, it's *never* too late to start!

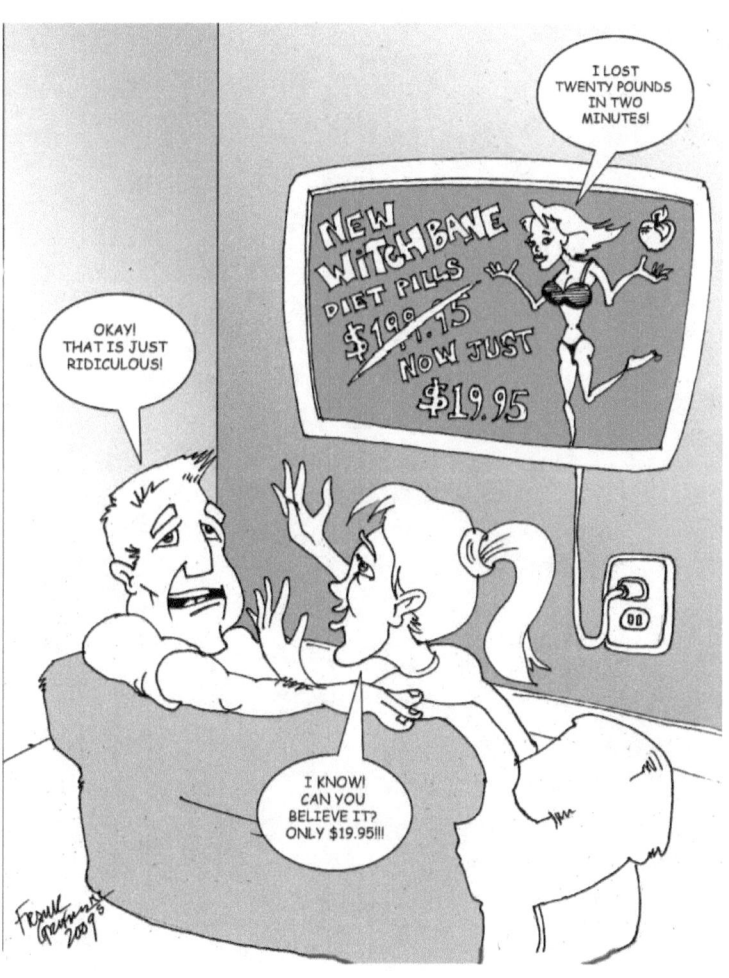

[123]

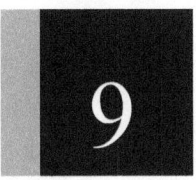

9

Will This Help Me Lose Weight or Not?
(Cut to the chase, buddy!)

There's no easy way to put this, outside of just coming out and saying, YES! Of course it will! It's not a quick fix, mind you. You won't be drinking a fluorescent orange liquid for two weeks and shedding thirty pounds, only to gain it back again the following month. You won't be jogging five times a day or going under the knife to have some suctioning done. No, this is a lifestyle change.

"Oh, great! What have a I gotten myself into?" you groan. Take heart. It's worth it. And, while it will be difficult at first, it will get easier . . . eventually. Trust me.

As with any major life change, especially one that may be reversing habits long embedded in our psyche, it's important to have a clear goal. We've talked a lot about what makes us happy. We've discovered that a life of giving is the one that's truly the most fulfilling. So, let's examine the goal within that. First, we need to ask ourselves: Are we trying the old "I'll-do-this-for-you-but-really-*me*-trickeroo?" Are we playing a little game here, changing our habits and our attitude toward focusing on others only because we think it will make *us* truly happy in the end?

It's like the little boy child who says he knows exactly what his younger, little sister wants for her birthday: a remote control monster tank that fires missiles and barks out army commands while crushing any toy in its path.

"She'll love it, really!" the boy says, pleadingly.

"Really?"

"Yes!"

"And you won't want to play with it at all? This is just for little Cindy?"

"Well, yeah, sure Dad. I mean, I might show her how to use it . . ."

"Her hands aren't even big enough to hold the remote control!"

"So, I'll hold it for her!"

Okay, obviously something's going on, there. And, I bring this up only to illustrate how sneaky our subconscious is. We are so used to looking out for *numero uno*, we might find ourselves doing it even if it looks like we're not. This is a self-examination I know I should take daily. For some darn reason and way too often, the selfish, "What can I get out of this?" attitude likes to sneak back into the forefront of my mind and then turn around and smile gloatingly in my face.

[126]

"You only agreed to bathe the little kids because you wanted to get permission to go play ball with the guys, didn't you? Didn't you!?"

"Whoah, take it easy."

"You're not fooling anyone, here. I know you. I am you! And we have to be in control, always scheming, planning, making sure we win in the end."

"Yeah, well, guess what? That was the old me. The new me is going to learn to simply . . . let go."

We are like skydivers, here. We need to jump into this life of love, trusting that the parachute will open when we need it to. So, take the dive. Feel the wind in your face, spread out your arms and try not to be afraid or doubt. The ground is not going to rush up at you and slap you in the face. Sure, it's going to be a bumpy ride, but I guarantee, the chute will open and you will soar gracefully through the heavens like an eagle. That kind of peace, no one and nothing can take away from you.

Jumping out of the plane won't be so hard, will it? Most of us are willing to *try* new things, especially if they carry a promise of a better life. The trick is staying with it. And, the trick to that is another tough word, especially in a society constantly peddling instant gratification: Patience.

We may have to fall for a long while before we feel the life-saving tug of that chute dragging us back into the clouds. But, it will come. We just need to hold on.

This is one of the major problems I find with most diets. They claim the world. "Slim those Winter Thighs

Just in Time for Spring!" "Get the Hot Body You Want Now!"

Now? Really? How does that work? Mail order? Body transplant? (I should watch what I say. Too many money-hungry scientists out there.) So, whether the diet inventor is realistic or not, we tend to expect great results within a relatively short amount of time.

"Hey, if I'm going to suffer like this, I better see some progress!"

"I went to bed hungry last night. I should be at least three pounds lighter this morning!"

Then, when we see that we're not making progress fast enough, we do a little math on the chalkboard of our minds: "Listen up class! We've seen less of the things we want going into our mouth area, but not enough leaving the buttocks and waist areas. The sacrifice is causing a great deal of pain in the cerebral area. So, let's see here: Less of what we want plus lots of pain and hardship equals . . . little results. Does that look right, class?! Oh, *no*! I don't think so! Time for a Pop Quiz on how many chocolates we can *pop* into our mouths in ten minutes! Better yet, let's make that a science experiment . . . "

When we don't see the pounds shedding right away, we tend to bail. Or, if the hardship we put ourselves through doesn't seem to be worth the benefit, we put on the brakes or swerve off the road into a river of indulgence. Again, like my grandmother used to say, "If you keep your expectations low, you'll never be disappointed." I don't think she meant expect little out of life or yourself. She was a wise woman, and I'm sure she was making the point that life is hard and the minute you are at peace with that, you can start seeing some silver linings. The moment we stop expecting to get everything we want, is the moment we start appreciating what we have.

So, what are you expecting out of this? "Yeah, I'll give it a shot. I'll start telling myself that food doesn't make me happy. I'll resist the urges, get through them, focus on others, take up sailing or sewing, but by gosh, if I don't fit into a size 12 by the end of the year I'm turning it all back around!"

Sounds a bit silly, huh?

See, the great thing about this plan of action is that you will see so many other great benefits and so many subtle and pure joys coming your way that it will seem nothing short of Midas-like foolishness to stop and go back to the way you were. Sure, like we just touched on, you're going to backslide at times and slip into moments of selfishness.

But, here is the real test. It will be your ability to get right back on track and keep moving forward that will prove the key to your success. And, the question at your darkest moment echoing in your mind will be, "Why? Why the heck am I doing this?"

What's your answer?

Because I want to be healthy so I can be around to enjoy my family in my old age?

So I can find fulfillment in life and help others do the same?

So I can be healthy and live as I was meant to live.

I'll take those. To me, these are solid goals. You don't see them plastered out there on billboards too often, do you? That's because the powers that be can't sell you a pill or anything else to make these things happen easily for you. It would be like seeing the following as ad slogans:

Life's hard. Get used to it.

Treat Yourself . . . to a life of sacrifice. It's worth it.

You Deserve Nothing Today. Give what you have to others.

Tough to read, huh? Kind of like "Love your neighbor as yourself." Like you love *yourself*. Wow, that's a lot of love. Or what about the good old toughie, "Love your enemies?" I bet the dairy farmers are gonna pick that one up any day now!

Milk. Love your enemies.

I can see it now.

So, why are you doing this? Why are you reading this book? Was it just for the fun of it? Was it just to get some new ideas that will get lost in the traffic jam of "to-do's," worries, "action items" and the millions of other thoughts crowding our minds every day?

It will be very easy to put this book down and get swallowed back into life again without a clear focus and a clear plan. It's great to detail a strategy: this is what I will eat at these times, this is what I can do as a hobby, and this is what I can do to help others, etc., but, to start, right now, just focus on your mission statement.

Ask yourself, "Why am I going to make these concrete changes in habit and attitude, finding true happiness in love and life, not food?" Now, write it in this space, right here. Writing something down is the first step to making it happen.

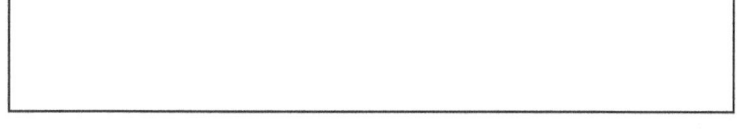

Now, mark this page. Remember it. Transcribe it to someplace you'll see every day, i.e., up on your mirror, inside your medicine cabinet, tattooed down your arm . . .

Bottom line of why *I'm* doing this? I know that, in the end, it will be better for me, my family and those in my life. And, as in so many other areas of pursuit, I need to remember that the destination can be found along the way. Let's not wait to be happy. Let's live it, now. If our heart's in the right place and we're trying to keep our mouths in line with it, then we can reach our goal every day.

We will see progress. We will feel better, healthier. It's not rocket science. We already know that, if we treat our body right, on a consistent basis, our body will treat *us* right.

Will weight be lost? Yes, if it needs to be, to get us to a healthy point of balance. Will people ask us to model underwear in our spare time? Probably not. Will we find

[131]

true fulfillment and make a difference in this world? I sincerely believe, <u>yes</u>.

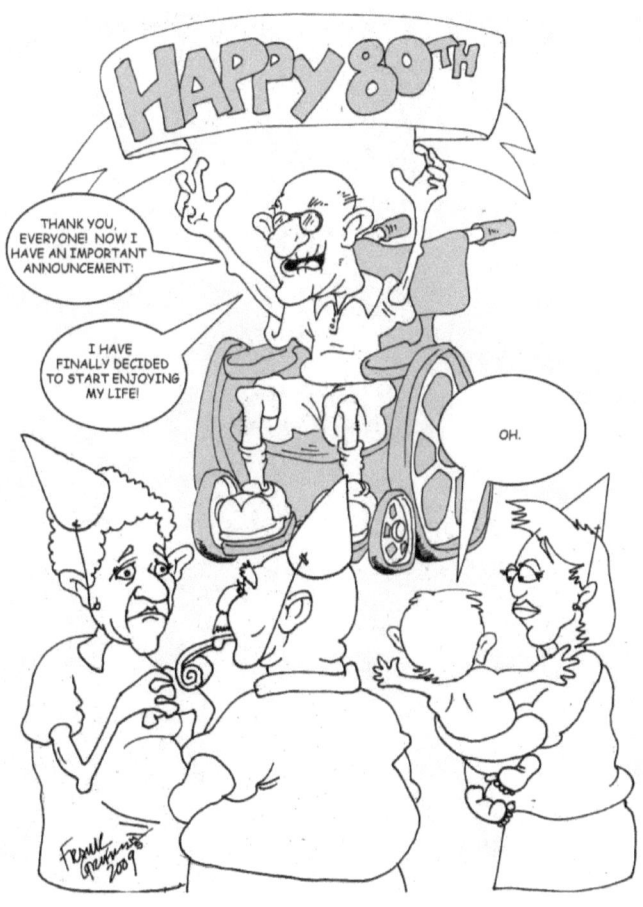

10

How's Your Relationship with Food Now?
(Some parting thoughts)

We started this journey together at the beginning of man's relationship with food. We've come down through my embarrassing years, taken a good look at where we're trying to find our happiness, and some ways we can attain joy and abstain from using food to get it. I hope it's been a beneficial venture for you. Here are some parting thoughts before you put this book down to eat something . . . healthy!

Parting Thought #1: Enjoy food. It's not the enemy. Unless, of course, you're talking about an enormous squid or great white shark. Then, yes, it could be considered an enemy. Lobsters? That depends. How many are we talking about, and are you in the tank with them?

Really, food was meant to taste good and be pleasurable. Only when we abuse it does it become something unhealthy. So, let's put food in its rightful place.

[135]

Yes, you guessed it, our mouths, moderately, and with the right perspective.

Parting Thought #2: <u>Enjoy life</u>! It's generally an all-around difficult experience, yes, but man, the perks are great. Don't lose sight of them. Live the way you were meant to live. Persevere and keep growing and learning, and you won't regret a moment of it. Don't hold back, thinking you'll live life once you look a certain way or feel a certain way. The time is now and it's not going to wait for you. *Carpe Diem. Seize the Day!*

And remember to be thankful. It's been said that a thankful heart is a happy heart. This is not just theoretical mishmash. It's literal truth. Even in my lowest moments, if I remember to, I can find a few solid things to be grateful for in my life and, almost immediately, I feel better. I know you can, too. Don't forget to lay this foundation every day of appreciating what you have. It's the key to true happiness.

How's your relationship with food now? Are you still infatuated with it? Do you love to hate it, hate to love it? Can you stand the sight of it? Can you at least be civil to it?

I hope you can pat a beef patty or shake hands with the nearest chicken drumstick and say, "Hey, you do your part and I'll do mine." Of course, don't make a habit of talking to your food, especially if you're in public.

Now get out there and enjoy food, live and love to the fullest, and be truly happy!

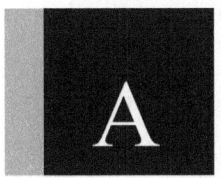

Appendix – Important Reminders

Here are some of the thoughts that we've touched on in the book that are worth repeating—over and over again. I'll list them here and then set them up as notes to cut out and place around your home, office, in your car, shower, refrigerator, or wherever they will serve to remind you of what you've gleaned from this book:

- ❖ My value is not based on how I look, but who I am.
- ❖ I am a work in progress. Priceless artwork.
- ❖ Food will not make me happy.
- ❖ Selfishness equals despair. Giving of myself equals true happiness.
- ❖ I can't do this alone.
- ❖ What's my hobby?
- ❖ I can solve world hunger.
- ❖ It's not about me.
- ❖ Food is not the enemy. Enjoy it.
- ❖ Enjoy life. Cherish each other.
- ❖ Moderation.

- ❖ Gosh, I love myself.
- ❖ Why am I doing this? What will my legacy be?
- ❖ Be who you are meant to be.
- ❖ Life's tough. Life well-lived is worth it.
- ❖ A Thankful Heart is a Happy Heart
- ❖ I'm thankful for what I have.
- ❖ Love to love.

My value is not based on how I look, but who I am.	I am a work in progress. Priceless artwork.
Food will <u>not</u> make me happy.	Selfishness = despair. Giving of myself = true happiness.
I can't do this alone.	What's my hobby?
I can solve world hunger.	It's not about me.

Food is not the enemy. Enjoy it.	*Enjoy life. Cherish each other.*
Moderation	Gosh, I love myself.
Why am I doing this? What will be my legacy?	Be who you are meant to be.
A Thankful Heart is a Happy Heart.	I'm thankful for what I have.
Life's tough. Life well-lived is worth it.	Love to love.

ABOUT THE AUTHOR

Michael Sortino has written scripts for film and television, as well as a handful of children's fiction and humor books. He's blessed with an understanding wife and four, adorable children, and yes, a healthy appetite as well! Feel free to contact him at michsort@gmail.com.

ABOUT THE ILLUSTRATOR

Frank Griffitts was born and raised most of his life in the Phoenix, Arizona area. He attributes his love for doodling and creativity to his friends, who were always encouraging and fun-loving. He currently resides in Arizona with his wife of more than 14 years and six kids. He works full time as a computer and video forensic analyst and helps his wife run a small video production company on the side. He is also heavily involved in his church and community where he currently serves as a counselor in the ward bishopric for The Church of Jesus Christ of Latter Day Saints.